Table of Contents

I0454200

The Palliative Care Nurse

The complete Guide

ALEXANDRE CAREWELL

Chapter 1:
Introduction to Palliative Care

Definitions and Basic Concepts

Origin and Evolution of the Term "Palliative

The term "palliative" has its origins in the Latin "pallium", meaning "cloak" or "veil". Through its linguistic evolution, the word has acquired a broader meaning in medicine, referring to an approach to care that aims to alleviate the symptoms and suffering of an illness without seeking a complete cure.

The use of the term "palliative" in the medical context dates back to ancient times, when Greek and Roman physicians already recognised the need to alleviate pain and relieve symptoms for patients in the advanced stages of incurable illnesses. However, it was only in the 20th century that the concept of palliative care gained in importance and recognition.
One of the major pioneers in the development of modern palliative care is Dame Cicely Saunders. A British doctor and social worker, she founded the first modern hospice in 1967, St. Christopher's Hospice in London. Saunders was one of the first to formalise the holistic approach to palliative care, emphasising pain management, emotional support, open communication and respect for the patient's dignity.

Over the decades, the concept of palliative care has continued to evolve, encompassing aspects such as patient-centred communication, shared decision-making and end-of-life care. Palliative care has also broadened its scope, affecting not only patients with advanced cancer, but also those with progressive chronic illnesses and a range of terminal conditions.

Today, palliative care has become an essential component of healthcare services, with growing recognition of the importance of providing patients with the best possible quality of life, even at the end of life. Palliative care is designed to meet the physical, psychological, social and spiritual needs of patients and their families, and it continues to evolve to adapt to medical advances and society's changing expectations.

The Transition from Curative to Palliative Care

The transition from curative to palliative care represents a crucial moment in the medical trajectory of a patient suffering from an incurable or terminal illness. This transition marks a paradigm shift from an approach focused on cure to one focused on symptom relief, quality of life and the patient's emotional well-being.

Curative care focuses on achieving a complete cure or remission of the disease. It often involves aggressive treatments such as surgery, chemotherapy and radiotherapy, with the aim of fighting the underlying disease. Sometimes, however, despite these treatments, the disease progresses or the treatment options are no longer effective.

It is at this stage that the transition to palliative care takes place. When the prospect of recovery diminishes, palliative care takes over to offer comprehensive support to the patient. The focus is on managing symptoms, preventing pain and discomfort, and improving quality of life. Palliative care aims to meet the physical, psychological, social and spiritual needs of patients and their families.

The transition to palliative care requires open and honest communication between the medical team, the patient and his or her family. Patients need to be informed in an understandable way about the course of their illness and the treatment options available. This enables patients to make informed decisions about their future care.

This transition can be an emotionally charged time for patients and their families. It can give rise to feelings of fear, anger and sadness, as well as concerns about the end of life. That's why palliative care healthcare professionals play a vital role in providing emotional support, answering questions and helping patients understand the benefits of palliative care.
Ultimately, the transition from curative to palliative care embodies the transition to an approach to care that focuses on quality of life, symptom relief and respect for the patient's values and choices. It marks the transition to a period when the patient's comfort, dignity and well-being are at the heart of medical care.

The Different Interpretations of Palliative Care

Palliative care, because of its holistic nature and patient-centred approach, can be interpreted in different ways depending on cultural, social and individual perspectives. These different interpretations reflect the complexity of each patient's needs and values, as well as the cultural and ethical influences that shape the understanding of palliative care around the world.

- **Relief of Pain and Suffering:** For many people, palliative care is primarily associated with the relief of physical pain and emotional suffering in patients who are terminally ill or suffering from incurable diseases. This interpretation emphasises the importance of providing maximum comfort to the patient while respecting their choices and dignity.
- **Improving quality of life:** Some people see palliative care as a way of improving the quality of life of patients at the end of life, by striving to minimise the side effects of treatment, prevent and manage symptoms, and promote a holistic approach that takes account of physical, emotional and social aspects.
- **Global Well-being Approach:** A broader interpretation of palliative care incorporates the notion of the patient's overall well-being, encompassing symptom management, psychological support, attention to spiritual needs and improved family relationships. This interpretation recognises the importance of treating the whole patient, beyond the illness.
- **Transition from curative treatments:** Palliative care can also be seen as a natural transition from intensive curative treatments to a gentler, patient-centred approach. This can involve a gradual shift from aggressive medical interventions to care aimed primarily at providing comfort and ensuring quality of life.
- **Respect for Values and Choices:** An ethical interpretation of palliative care emphasises absolute respect for the patient's values and choices. It aims to honour the patient's wishes at the end of life, whether these involve refusing aggressive treatment or seeking a peaceful and comfortable end to life.
- **Family support:** Palliative care also encompasses support for families and loved ones, recognising the emotional impact of terminal illness on everyone around the patient.

These different interpretations reflect the diversity of perspectives on palliative care, while highlighting its adaptable and flexible nature to meet the specific needs of each individual and their family. This diversity also reflects the complexity of the ethical, cultural and psychological issues surrounding the end of life and the care of terminally ill patients.

Philosophy and Objectives of Palliative Care

Relieving Suffering rather than Healing
One of the fundamental principles of palliative care is that the primary goal is not to cure the underlying disease, but rather to relieve suffering and improve the quality of life of patients in the advanced stages or at the end of life. This approach is based on the recognition that, in some cases, complete cure is not possible and that patients face unique physical, emotional and spiritual challenges.

Palliative care takes a holistic view of the patient. Rather than concentrating on suppressing the disease, it focuses on managing symptoms, relieving pain, preventing discomfort and improving quality of life. This approach aims to enable patients to live as comfortably and actively as possible, while respecting their wishes and choices regarding treatment and the end of life. The fundamental idea behind this approach is that each patient is unique, with individual needs and values. Therefore, the palliative care team works with the patient and family to develop a personalised care plan that meets each person's specific needs. This involves open discussions about goals of care, treatment options and personal preferences.

The relief of suffering in palliative care encompasses not only the management of physical pain, but also addressing the emotional, social and spiritual aspects of suffering. Patients at the end of life may experience feelings of anxiety, fear, sadness and loss of control. Palliative care aims to offer emotional and psychological support, as well as facilitating conversations about important issues such as end-of-life wishes and comfort care.

This approach, which focuses on relieving suffering, can have a significant impact on patients' quality of life and their experience of the end of life. It allows patients to focus on what is important to them, to create precious memories with their loved ones and to live each day with dignity and respect. By emphasising compassion, empathy and attentive listening, palliative care honours the value of every life, even when a full recovery is no longer a realistic option.

The Holistic Approach to the Patient at the End of Life
The holistic approach is at the heart of palliative care, guiding the care of patients at the end of life in a way that recognises and responds to their complex and multidimensional nature. This approach views the patient as a whole being, integrating the physical, psychological, social and spiritual aspects of their existence. It aims to provide comprehensive support that goes beyond mere medical treatment, offering patients the opportunity to live out their final days with dignity, comfort and respect.

- **Physical:** The holistic approach takes into account the physical needs of the patient at the end of life. This includes pain management, prevention and treatment of symptoms such as fatigue, nausea and dyspnoea (difficulty breathing). Palliative care focuses on maintaining an optimal level of comfort for the patient, adapting treatments to minimise side effects and promoting physical well-being.
- **Psychological aspect:** Patients at the end of life can face emotional challenges such as anxiety, depression, fear and loss of control. The holistic approach aims to offer psychological and emotional support, providing a safe space to express feelings and concerns. Palliative care healthcare professionals are trained to listen with compassion, offer support and help patients cope with their emotions.
- **Social aspect:** Social and family relationships play an essential role in the lives of patients at the end of life. The holistic approach integrates family and loved ones into patient care, providing support to maintain meaningful relationships and facilitating communication between family members. Palliative care recognises the importance of the patient's social support network and strives to strengthen it.

- **Spiritual aspect:** The spiritual dimension can be profoundly important for many patients at the end of life, whether they have a religious belief or not. Palliative care respects the spiritual dimension of the patient, offering time for reflection, prayer or meditation according to individual preferences and beliefs. This dimension helps to bring meaning and peace of mind to patients at the end of life.

The holistic approach to the patient at the end of life is the essence of palliative care, reflecting the recognition of the complexity of each individual and their diverse needs. By addressing the physical, psychological, social and spiritual aspects of the patient, palliative care aims to improve quality of life, reduce suffering and honour the dignity and worth of each person during this delicate phase of their journey.

Maintaining Quality of Life and Dignity

Maintaining quality of life and dignity is one of the cornerstones of palliative care. When complete cure is no longer a realistic option, palliative care focuses on creating an environment where patients at the end of life can live their remaining days with comfort, respect and optimal quality of life, while preserving their dignity and autonomy.

- **Symptom Management:** Painful and uncomfortable symptoms are common in patients at the end of life. Palliative care focuses on identifying, assessing and effectively managing these symptoms to improve the patient's physical comfort. This may involve the use of medication, complementary therapies and pain management techniques to ensure maximum relief.
- **Preservation of autonomy:** Patients at the end of life may feel a loss of control over their lives as the disease progresses. Palliative care places a strong emphasis on respecting patients' autonomy. Healthcare professionals work closely with patients to determine their wishes regarding treatment, to give them the opportunity to make informed decisions about their care and to respect their personal choices.
- **Personalised Care Planning:** An individualised approach to palliative care means that each patient has a care plan tailored to their specific needs. Palliative care healthcare professionals work with the patient and family

to develop a care plan that takes into account the patient's wishes, treatment preferences and overall needs.

- **Emotional and Psychological Support:** Patients at the end of life can experience a complex range of emotions, from anxiety to sadness to anger. Palliative care offers emotional and psychological support to help patients cope with these feelings, express their concerns and find ways to live with a positive outlook despite their circumstances.
- **Maintaining Family Relationships:** The end of life can be a time when family relationships are put to the test. Palliative care encourages open communication between the patient, family and loved ones. It offers support in maintaining meaningful relationships, easing conflicts and creating precious memories.
- **Respect for Dignity:** Patient dignity is a fundamental principle of palliative care. Palliative care healthcare professionals recognise the intrinsic value of each individual and ensure that the patient is treated with respect, compassion and dignity at all times.

In short, maintaining quality of life and dignity is at the heart of the palliative care philosophy. By offering comprehensive support that takes into account the physical, emotional, social and spiritual aspects of a patient's life, palliative care aims to create an environment where each patient can live out their final days in a meaningful and comfortable way, while preserving their dignity and autonomy.

History of Palliative Care

The Pioneers of Palliative Care : Dame Cicely Saunders

Dame Cicely Saunders is widely recognised as one of the major pioneers in the development and promotion of modern palliative care. Her ground-breaking work and passion for improving the quality of life of patients in the late stages of life and at the end of life laid the foundations for what has become an essential and respectful approach to care.

Born on 22 June 1918 in England, Cicely Saunders was both a doctor and a social worker. She began her career in nursing and went on to study medicine at the age of 33. It was during her work as a medical student that she was deeply affected by the experience of terminally ill patients in a London hospice.

Saunders was struck by the lack of specialist care and support for patients at the end of life, which motivated her quest to create an environment where patients could live out their final days with dignity and comfort. In 1967, she founded St. Christopher's Hospice, the first modern hospice in London. It was an innovative place that incorporated a holistic approach to palliative care.

Cicely Saunders' approach to palliative care was deeply humane and holistic. She firmly believed in the need to relieve physical pain, but she also understood the importance of meeting patients' emotional, psychological and spiritual needs. She introduced the concept of 'total pain', which encompasses all the suffering associated with terminal illness, including physical pain, emotional pain, psychological suffering and spiritual needs. Cicely Saunders' vision has also helped to educate healthcare professionals in palliative care, emphasising the importance of attentive listening, open communication and empathy towards patients at the end of life. Her influence extended far beyond the UK, inspiring the creation of hospices and palliative care programmes around the world.

Dame Cicely Saunders has left a lasting legacy in the field of palliative care. Her dedication to improving the quality of life for patients at the end of life, her emphasis on dignity, respect and a holistic approach to care have influenced the way palliative care is delivered today. She laid the foundations for a patient-centred approach that recognises the value and importance of every life, even at the most difficult times.

The Evolution of Palliative Care Worldwide

The evolution of palliative care worldwide reflects a significant transformation in the way society approaches the end of life, pain and suffering. While palliative care has historical roots, its development and official recognition as a medical discipline in its own right have been marked by significant progress in recent decades.

In the early stages of the palliative care movement, pioneers such as Dame Cicely Saunders laid the foundations of the modern approach by focusing on the relief of suffering, pain management and quality of life for terminally ill patients. St. Christopher's Hospice, founded by Saunders, became the model for many other hospices around the world.

However, it has taken time for palliative care to be fully recognised and integrated into healthcare systems. Over the years, thanks to the efforts of activists, health professionals and international organisations, palliative care has gained in visibility and importance. Here are some key milestones in the development of palliative care worldwide:

- **1970s-1980s: Expansion of Hospices and Palliative Care Programmes**
  The 1970s and 1980s saw a rapid growth in the number of hospices and palliative care programmes around the world, largely as a result of the growing recognition of the importance of treating patients at the end of life holistically.
- **1990s: Training and Education for Health Professionals**
  During the 1990s, palliative care training and education programmes were developed for healthcare professionals. This helped to raise the quality of palliative care and train a new generation of specialist practitioners.
- **2000s: International recognition**
  In the early 2000s, the World Health Organisation (WHO) recognised palliative care as an essential component of health services. This led to greater integration of palliative care into national and international health policies.
- **2010 and Beyond: Expanding Areas of Application**
  Over the past decade, palliative care has broadened its scope to include not only terminally ill cancer patients, but also those with chronic progressive diseases, heart disease, dementia and other conditions. Paediatric palliative care has also gained in importance.
- **Integration into health systems**
  More and more countries are integrating palliative care into their healthcare systems, providing greater access to palliative care for patients and families. Multidisciplinary palliative care teams work alongside medical teams to provide comprehensive support.

The evolution of palliative care worldwide shows a growing recognition of the importance of preserving the dignity, quality of life and comfort of patients at the end of life. Palliative care is now considered an essential part of healthcare, with constant progress in research, training and integration into national healthcare systems.

Recognition and legitimacy of palliative care

The recognition and legitimacy of palliative care have evolved significantly over the years, from a marginal approach to an essential medical discipline integrated into healthcare systems around the world. This evolution reflects a growing awareness of the importance of preserving the dignity, quality of life and well-being of terminally ill and dying patients.

- **From Marginalisation to Recognition:** Initially, palliative care was often seen as an alternative and marginal approach to aggressive curative treatments. However, thanks to the efforts of pioneers such as Dame Cicely Saunders and the demonstration of the effectiveness of palliative care in relieving pain and suffering, it has gained recognition.
- **Integration into healthcare systems: Over the** last few decades, palliative care has gained legitimacy by being gradually integrated into national healthcare systems. Health organisations and governments have recognised that palliative care is a complementary and essential approach to curative treatments, offering comprehensive support to patients at the end of life.
- **Recognition by the World Health   Organisation (WHO):** In 2002, the WHO published its report on palliative care, recognising its importance as a vital component of health services. This international recognition has helped to strengthen the position of palliative care in the medical field and to encourage governments to integrate palliative care into their health policies.
- **Training and education:** The legitimacy of palliative care has also been strengthened by the development of training and education programmes for healthcare professionals. Universities and medical institutions now offer specialist programmes in palliative care, training a new generation of competent practitioners.
- **Research and evidence:** Palliative care research has helped to establish a solid basis for the legitimacy of this approach. Clinical studies and research into the effects of palliative care on quality of life, pain management and patient satisfaction have reinforced its credibility.

16

- **Patient and Family Support: The** positive experience of patients and their families who have benefited from quality palliative care has played an important role in the recognition and legitimacy of this care. Testimonials and positive feedback have demonstrated the positive impact of palliative care on the lives of patients at the end of life.

The growing recognition and legitimacy of palliative care testifies to its importance as an essential medical approach. Palliative care has evolved into a multidisciplinary discipline that is integrated into healthcare systems, addressing the physical, emotional, social and spiritual needs of patients at the end of life and their families.

The place of palliative care in the medical field

Palliative care complements curative treatment
Palliative care and curative treatments are two distinct approaches to medical care, but they can be complementary and interact in a way that is beneficial for patients with serious or terminal illnesses. While curative treatments aim to combat the underlying disease, palliative care focuses on relieving pain and suffering and improving quality of life. The complementary nature of these two approaches can provide comprehensive, holistic care for patients.

- **Different Goals, Overall Coherence:** Curative treatments aim to eradicate the disease, while palliative care focuses on managing symptoms and improving quality of life, even when complete cure is not possible. The two approaches can coexist in coherence, where curative treatments can be continued while integrating palliative care to improve patient comfort.
- **Managing side effects:** Curative treatments such as chemotherapy and radiotherapy can often lead to unwanted side effects such as nausea, fatigue and loss of appetite. Palliative care can play an essential role in managing these side effects, ensuring that patients can tolerate treatment and maintain an optimal quality of life.
- **Gradual transition:** As the disease progresses and curative treatment options become less effective, palliative care can be introduced gradually to help the patient make

a smooth transition from a healing approach to one focused on comfort and quality of life.

- **Emotional Support:** Curative treatments can be emotionally challenging for patients and their families. Palliative care offers emotional and psychological support to help patients cope with the anxiety, fear and stress associated with treatment and illness.
- **Holistic Care:** Together, palliative care and curative treatments can provide holistic care for the patient. Palliative care health professionals work closely with the medical team to ensure that the patient's physical, emotional and spiritual needs are taken into account.
- **Support for loved ones:** Palliative care also provides support for loved ones and families, helping them to navigate the emotional and practical challenges of illness and treatment.

Ultimately, the complementarity of palliative care with curative treatments can provide more holistic, patient-centred care. This approach recognises the multiple needs of patients with serious or terminal illnesses and aims to improve their quality of life while maintaining a balance between treating the underlying illness and relieving pain and suffering.

Advances in Palliative Medicine over time
Palliative medicine has undergone significant advances over time, resulting from a combination of medical progress, clinical research, increased awareness and a better understanding of the needs of patients at the end of life. These advances have helped to transform palliative care into a medical discipline that is respected, recognised and widely integrated into healthcare systems around the world.

- **Pain and symptom management:** One of the most significant advances in palliative care has been the development of advanced pain and symptom management techniques. More effective drugs, innovative approaches to pain management and complementary therapies have been developed to offer patients optimal relief.
- **Individualised Care Plans:** With the emphasis on a holistic approach, palliative care has evolved towards more individualised care plans. Palliative care healthcare professionals work closely with patients and their families

to create personalised care plans that meet their specific needs and values.

- **Paediatric palliative care: A** significant advance has been the recognition of the importance of paediatric palliative care for children with serious and terminal illnesses. Palliative care for children has become a distinct speciality, taking into account the unique needs of young patients and their families.
- **Palliative care research :** Research in palliative care has developed considerably, contributing to a better understanding of patients' needs and the development of best practice. Clinical studies have evaluated the effectiveness of palliative care treatments and interventions, guiding practitioners towards evidence-based approaches.
- **Training and Education:** The establishment of specialised training and education programmes in palliative care has resulted in the training of highly qualified healthcare professionals in this field. Multidisciplinary training has strengthened the skills of palliative care teams and helped to ensure high-quality care.
- **Integration into health systems: The** growing integration of palliative care into national and regional health systems is a major step forward. More and more countries are recognising palliative care as an essential component of health services and integrating it into their health policies.
- **Technological advances:** Technological advances have also contributed to palliative care. Telecare, symptom-tracking applications and online communication tools make it easier to monitor patients and access palliative care, even at a distance.

The constant evolution of palliative care is a testament to the discipline's ability to adapt to the changing needs of patients and medical advances. These advances have improved the quality of life of patients at the end of life, increased awareness of the importance of palliative care and ensured that patients receive the most appropriate and compassionate care possible.

Palliative Care as a Fundamental Right of the Patient

Palliative care has become increasingly recognised not only as an essential medical approach, but also as a fundamental right of the patient at the end of life. Addressing the physical,

19

emotional, social and spiritual needs of terminally ill patients reflects a holistic view of human dignity and respect for life, and is an inherent right of every individual.

- **Right to Dignity and Comfort:** Terminally ill patients have the right to live out their final days in dignity and comfort. Palliative care aims to relieve pain and symptoms, offer emotional support and improve quality of life, ensuring that every patient is treated with respect and compassion.
- **Right to Autonomy and Choice:** Patients have the right to participate in decisions about their care and treatment. Palliative care emphasises the principle of patient autonomy, providing full information about treatment options, respecting personal choice and involving patients in planning their care.
- **Right to Communication and Information:** Patients have the right to be informed in an understandable way about their condition, their treatment options and the implications of these choices. Palliative care health professionals promote open and honest communication to enable patients to make informed decisions.
- **Right to Spirituality and Beliefs:** Palliative care recognises patients' right to express their spirituality and beliefs, whether religious or not. Respect for the patient's spiritual dimension is fundamental to providing comprehensive and holistic support.
- **Right to Quality of Life:** Every patient has the right to live a quality life, even in the terminal phase. Palliative care strives to improve quality of life by taking into account the patient's physical, emotional, social and spiritual needs.
- **The right to personalised care:** Patients have the right to receive care that is tailored to their individual needs and preferences. Palliative care focuses on creating personalised care plans that take into account the patient's values and wishes.
- **The right to family and loved ones:** Patients have the right to be surrounded by their loved ones and to receive family support during the terminal phase. Palliative care recognises the importance of social and family support
- and often includes families in its care.

The recognition of palliative care as a fundamental patient right reflects a major advance in the way society views the end of life.

This approach emphasises the values of compassion, respect and dignity, and ensures that each individual can live out their final days according to their preferences and needs, surrounded by a team of healthcare professionals committed to providing compassionate, high-quality care.

Importance of Palliative Care in Society

Demographic challenges and an ageing population
Demographic change, characterised by an ageing population, poses significant challenges for palliative care. With life expectancy increasing and populations ageing in many parts of the world, it is becoming imperative to develop appropriate approaches to meet the growing needs of the terminally ill and the dying.

- **Population ageing:** Increased life expectancy, combined with lower birth rates, is leading to an increase in the proportion of elderly people in the population. This demographic trend is particularly visible in industrialised countries and poses challenges in terms of meeting the specific needs of this population.
- **Complex Medical Conditions:** Elderly people often present with a multitude of chronic and complex health problems, such as heart disease, neurological conditions and degenerative diseases. Managing these terminal conditions requires a multidisciplinary approach and a thorough understanding of medical interactions.
- **Growing need for palliative care:** The ageing of the population is leading to an increase in the number of people requiring palliative care. Palliative care resources will therefore need to be expanded to meet growing demand.
- **Complex Social and Emotional Needs:** Terminally ill older people can face unique social and emotional challenges, such as isolation, loneliness and concern for loved ones. Palliative care must take these aspects into account to provide holistic support.
- **End-of-Life Preferences:** Older people may have specific preferences regarding their care at the end of life, including the place of death. Palliative care must be able to respect these preferences while providing quality care.

- **Specialised training:** Healthcare professionals will need to be trained to deal with the particular needs of terminally ill older people. This includes an understanding of the medical conditions associated with ageing and the skills to communicate with elderly patients and their families.
- **Burden on families:** The ageing of the population can also increase the burden on families and carers, who often provide care for the terminally ill. Palliative care must include support for families and informal carers.

Responding to demographic challenges and an ageing population requires a proactive and considered approach to palliative care. It is crucial to develop strategies to anticipate future needs, to expand palliative care resources and to put in place care systems that recognise and take account of age-related specificities in the care of patients at the end of life.

Reducing medical costs through palliative care

Palliative care plays an important role in reducing the medical costs associated with aggressive treatments at the end of life. By adopting an approach focused on pain relief, quality of life and symptom management, palliative care can help reduce the expense of unnecessary or inappropriate treatments, while offering holistic support to patients and their families.

- **Avoidance of Unnecessary Treatments:** Terminally ill patients who no longer benefit from aggressive curative treatments may be subjected to costly and potentially harmful medical interventions. Palliative care focuses on providing care that corresponds to the patient's needs and wishes, thus avoiding unnecessary and costly treatments.
- **Reducing repeat hospitalisations:** Terminally ill patients can experience costly multiple hospital admissions. Palliative care at home or in a hospice can help manage symptoms and provide medical and emotional support, reducing the need for frequent hospitalisations.
- **Optimising Use of Resources:** Palliative care uses resources efficiently by targeting interventions on what matters most to the patient. This optimises the use of hospital beds, medical staff and equipment.
- **Better pain management:** Effective pain and symptom management reduces the need for costly medical

interventions to treat the side effects of aggressive treatments.

- **Reduction in terminal treatments:** Aggressive curative treatments in the terminal phase may not offer significant benefits and can be costly. Palliative care focuses on the needs of the patient and can reduce reliance on ineffective treatments.
- **Promoting home care:** Palliative care at home can be a more affordable alternative to hospitalisation, while offering a comfortable and familiar environment for the patient.
- **Improved Quality of Life:** By improving quality of life and reducing pain and suffering, patients can have a more positive experience at the end of life, which can also have a positive impact on the associated mental and emotional health costs.
- **Early Care Planning:** Early palliative care planning enables patients and their families to make informed decisions and avoid unnecessary expenditure at the end of life.

By adopting a patient-centred approach and focusing on quality of life and effective symptom management, palliative care can not only improve the patient's experience at the end of life, but also contribute to significant savings in medical costs. This holistic approach promotes a more efficient use of resources while offering patients compassionate care that respects their needs and wishes.

Palliative Care in a Cultural and Religious Context

Palliative care must take into account the cultural and religious diversity of patients at the end of life, recognising the importance of their beliefs, values and practices in the care process. Respect for these cultural and religious aspects is essential to providing quality care that is respectful and adapted to the individual needs of patients and their families.

- **Cultural diversity:** Patients at the end of life come from different cultures, each with its own norms, traditions and values. Palliative care needs to be sensitive to this diversity and adapt care approaches according to cultural beliefs and specific practices.

- **Importance of Communication:** Healthcare professionals in palliative care need to establish open and respectful communication with patients and their families to understand their cultural and religious beliefs. This allows care to be personalised by taking these factors into account.
- **Funeral practices:** Funeral practices vary from one culture to another. It is important to respect the wishes of the patient and his or her family with regard to funeral rituals and preparations after death.
- **Spiritual rites :** Palliative care must allow patients and their families to practise their spiritual rites and rituals in accordance with their religious beliefs.
- **Food and dietary restrictions:** Some religious beliefs impose dietary restrictions or specific standards for food preparation. Palliative care must respect these nutritional needs while providing meals that are compatible with religious prescriptions.
- **Spiritual care:** The spiritual and religious needs of patients at the end of life must be taken into account. Palliative care should offer spiritual or religious support according to the patient's preferences.
- **Families and communities:** Palliative care often involves the patient's family and community. It is important to understand family dynamics and cultural roles in order to provide appropriate support.
- **Cultural and Religious Training:** Health professionals in palliative care must be trained to recognise and respect the cultural and religious needs of patients. Awareness and education are essential to providing appropriate care.
- **Interdisciplinary collaboration:** Social workers, spiritual advisers and other professionals can play an important role in addressing the cultural and religious aspects of palliative care. Interdisciplinary collaboration is essential to provide comprehensive care.

Palliative care in a cultural and religious context requires a flexible and respectful approach that recognises the individual needs of patients and their families. By integrating cultural and religious beliefs and practices into care planning, palliative care can offer comprehensive care that respects the dignity and values of every patient at the end of life.

Chapter 2:
Fundamental Principles of Palliative Care

Global and Holistic Approach to the Patient

Taking account of physical, psychological and social needs

Palliative care takes a holistic approach that recognises the multiple and interconnected needs of patients at the end of life. This comprehensive approach takes into account physical, psychological and social needs, aiming to improve quality of life and offer comprehensive support to patients and their families.

- **Physical needs:** Patients at the end of life may experience a range of physical symptoms and pain, such as pain, fatigue, nausea and dyspnoea. Palliative care healthcare professionals assess and manage these symptoms effectively to reduce suffering and improve patient comfort.
- **Psychological needs:** Patients at the end of life may experience a range of emotions, including anxiety, fear, sadness and distress. Palliative care provides psychological and emotional support to help patients cope with these emotions and improve their mental well-being.
- **Social needs:** Patients at the end of life may experience isolation and loneliness, and their social needs must also be taken into account. Palliative care encourages family and social support, facilitates interaction with friends and relatives, and helps patients maintain their social ties.
- **Spiritual support:** For some patients, spiritual and religious needs are important at the end of life. Palliative care recognises these needs and provides spiritual or religious support according to the patient's preferences.
- **Quality of life: The** ultimate aim of palliative care is to improve the patient's quality of life. This involves understanding the physical, psychological and social aspects that contribute to quality of life and working to optimise them.
- **Personalised approach:** Every patient has unique needs. Palliative care healthcare professionals work with

patients and their families to create personalised care plans that meet their specific needs.

- **Open Communication:** Open communication between patients, families and healthcare professionals is essential to identify and respond to physical, psychological and social needs. Open communication also allows patients to voice their concerns and preferences.
- **Multidisciplinary team:** Palliative care often involves a multidisciplinary team of doctors, nurses, social workers, spiritual advisers and other professionals. This team works together to provide comprehensive care that takes into account all aspects of the patient's needs.

By taking into account the physical, psychological and social needs of patients at the end of life, palliative care offers a holistic approach that aims to improve quality of life, relieve suffering and provide comprehensive support. This holistic approach recognises the importance of treating each patient as an individual, with unique needs and preferences.

Individualised Care Based on Patient Personality
An essential component of palliative care is the individualisation of care according to the patient's personality. Each patient is unique, with his or her own personality, preferences and values. Palliative care professionals recognise the importance of this individuality and tailor care to meet the specific needs of each patient.

- **In-depth assessment:** Individualised care begins with an in-depth assessment of the patient's personality, preferences and values. Palliative care health professionals take the time to get to know the patient and understand what matters most to them.
- **Respecting preferences:** Palliative care takes into account the patient's preferences in terms of treatment, symptom management and decision-making. Healthcare professionals work with patients to respect their choices and wishes.
- **Adapting communication:** Communication with patients is adapted according to their personality. Some patients may prefer detailed information, while others may prefer more concise and gentle communication.

26

- **Compassionate approach:** Palliative care recognises that each patient is unique and requires a compassionate and individualised approach. Palliative care health professionals strive to create a bond with the patient to better understand their needs and offer appropriate support.
- **Incorporating hobbies and interests:** Palliative care can incorporate the patient's hobbies and interests into care planning. This can help to maintain quality of life and create moments of joy.
- **Personalised psychological support:** Patients react differently to illness and the end of life, depending on their personality. Palliative care healthcare professionals offer personalised psychological support to help patients deal with their emotions and concerns.
- **Family collaboration:** Individualising care often involves collaboration with the patient's family. Relatives are familiar with the patient's personality and can help to personalise care.
- **Maintaining dignity:** Individualised care helps to maintain the patient's dignity. Care is adapted to respect the patient's personality and wishes.

Individualising care according to the patient's personality reflects palliative care's commitment to treating each patient as a unique person, with their own needs, values and preferences. By taking into account the patient's personality, palliative care creates a respectful, compassionate and patient-centred care environment, thereby promoting a more positive and satisfying end-of-life experience.

Interdisciplinary Collaboration for a Global Approach

Interdisciplinary collaboration is at the heart of palliative care, enabling a holistic and comprehensive approach to meet the complex needs of patients at the end of life. Professionals from different disciplines work together to provide holistic care that encompasses physical, psychological, social and spiritual aspects, while ensuring effective coordination and transparent communication.

- **Multidisciplinary team:** Palliative care usually involves a multidisciplinary team of doctors, nurses, social workers, spiritual advisors, therapists and other health professionals. Each member of the team brings unique expertise to offer comprehensive care.

- **Transparent communication:** Interdisciplinary collaboration relies on transparent and regular communication between team members. This allows relevant information to be shared, care to be coordinated and treatment plans to be adjusted according to the patient's needs.
- **Coherent Care Planning:** By working together, palliative care healthcare professionals develop coherent care plans that take into account all aspects of the patient's needs. This avoids redundancies and ensures efficient use of resources.
- **Holistic approach:** Each professional brings expertise in their respective field, contributing to a comprehensive and holistic approach. For example, nurses may focus on physical needs, social workers on social and emotional aspects, and spiritual counsellors on spiritual needs.
- **Emotional support:** The emotions and concerns of patients at the end of life require special attention. Interdisciplinary collaboration enables emotional support to be provided more comprehensively, helping patients to cope with their worries and emotions.
- **Comprehensive care:** Palliative care aims to provide comprehensive care. Interdisciplinary collaboration enables all the patient's needs to be met, ensuring that no important aspect is overlooked.
- **Personalised approach:** By working together, the interdisciplinary team can tailor care to the patient's individual needs and preferences. This helps to improve quality of life and patient satisfaction.
- **Continuing education:** Health professionals working in palliative care need to be continually trained and keep abreast of developments in their respective fields. Interdisciplinary collaboration encourages continuous learning and the updating of knowledge.

Interdisciplinary collaboration is a cornerstone of palliative care, ensuring a holistic, comprehensive and patient-centred approach. By working together, palliative care healthcare professionals are better equipped to meet the complex and varied needs of patients at the end of life, providing comprehensive support that improves quality of life and brings comfort to patients and their families.

Pain and Suffering Relief

Differentiating between Physical Pain and Emotional Suffering

In palliative care, it is crucial to distinguish between physical pain and emotional suffering, as they are two distinct but interconnected aspects of patients' well-being at the end of life. Understanding the difference between these two concepts enables healthcare professionals to provide effective relief and comprehensive care.

- **Physical pain:** Physical pain is a sensory and subjective experience that results from the activation of nerve receptors in response to a nociceptive stimulus. It can be localised or generalised and can be described in terms of quality (e.g. stabbing, burning, oppressive), intensity (mild, moderate, severe) and duration (acute, chronic).
- **Pain assessment:** Health professionals in palliative care use pain assessment tools to determine the nature and intensity of physical pain. This enables analgesic treatments to be adapted and the patient's response to care to be monitored.
- **Pain Management:** Physical pain management involves the use of analgesics and non-pharmacological techniques to relieve pain. Medication, physical therapies, massage and relaxation techniques can be used to alleviate physical pain.
- **Emotional Suffering:** Emotional suffering encompasses a range of negative emotions such as anxiety, fear, sadness, anger and despair. Unlike physical pain, emotional suffering is linked to the psychological and affective aspects of the patient's experience at the end of life.
- **Assessing emotional distress:** Assessing emotional distress requires open and empathic communication between healthcare professionals and patients. Patients can express their emotions, concerns and fears that contribute to their emotional suffering.
- **Psychological support:** Managing emotional suffering involves psychological and emotional support. Palliative care healthcare professionals can offer attentive listening, advice, supportive therapies and interventions to help patients cope with their emotions.

- **Holistic approach:** A holistic approach recognises the interconnection between physical pain and emotional suffering. Effective relief of physical pain can also help to reduce emotional suffering, and vice versa.
- **Open communication:** Palliative care healthcare professionals should encourage patients to communicate openly about their physical pain and emotions. This helps to provide holistic care and ensures that all aspects of suffering are addressed.

Distinguishing between physical pain and emotional suffering is essential for comprehensive and effective care of patients at the end of life. Palliative care healthcare professionals use their expertise to assess and treat both aspects appropriately, ensuring that patients receive effective relief and comprehensive management of their physical and emotional needs.

Use of Pain Assessment Scales
Pain assessment is a fundamental stage in the management of palliative care patients. Pain assessment scales are clinical tools used to measure the intensity of pain experienced by patients. They enable palliative care healthcare professionals to obtain objective information about the patient's pain, personalise analgesic treatments and monitor the effectiveness of interventions.

- **Assessment objective:** Pain assessment scales aim to quantify a patient's pain in order to obtain objective data to guide treatment decisions. This makes it possible to monitor changes in pain over time and adjust interventions accordingly.
- **Types of scales:** There are several types of pain assessment scales, ranging from simple numerical scales to more detailed verbal or graphical scales. Patients may be asked to rate their pain on a scale from 0 to 10, to choose words to describe their pain (such as "no pain", "mild pain", "moderate pain", "severe pain"), or to indicate the location of the pain on a body chart.
- **Appropriate choice:** The choice of scale depends on the patient's ability and preference. Simple scales are more suitable for patients who are able to communicate verbally, while graphic scales may be more appropriate for patients who have difficulty expressing themselves verbally.

- **Frequency of Assessment:** Pain assessment should be carried out regularly and systematically. The frequency may vary depending on the clinical situation, but should be sufficient to monitor changes in the patient's pain.
- **Continuous assessment:** Health professionals in palliative care must maintain a continuous assessment of pain throughout the period of care. Pain can change with treatment, disease progression and other factors.
- **Inclusion of Patient Preferences:** When assessing pain, it is important to take into account the patient's preferences for pain treatment and management. This allows interventions to be tailored to what is most important to the patient.
- **Open communication:** Palliative care healthcare professionals should encourage patients to communicate openly about their pain and to use assessment scales as tools for expressing their feelings.
- **Staff training:** Palliative care healthcare professionals must be trained in the appropriate use of pain assessment scales to ensure accurate and reliable measurements.

The use of pain assessment scales in palliative care improves communication between patients and healthcare professionals, enabling more targeted and effective pain management. These scales also help to individualise care by adapting treatments to the specific needs of each patient, thereby improving quality of life and comfort at the end of life.

Multimodal Approaches to Pain Management
Pain management in palliative care is often based on multimodal approaches, which combine different interventions to achieve effective and complete pain relief. These approaches recognise that pain at the end of life can be complex and varied, requiring a combination of treatments to meet the patient's individual needs.

- **Combination of therapies:** Multimodal approaches involve combining pharmacological and non-pharmacological treatments to target different aspects of pain. Analgesics, physical therapies, relaxation techniques and psychological approaches can be used together.

- **Personalised treatment:** Every patient reacts differently to pain and to treatments. Multimodal approaches make it possible to tailor treatments to the patient's specific needs, targeting the aspects of pain that have the greatest impact on their quality of life.
- **More effective relief:** By combining several treatments, multimodal approaches offer more effective pain relief by acting on several pain transmission pathways. This can reduce the need for high doses of analgesics and minimise side effects.
- **Reducing side effects:** Pharmacological treatments can have undesirable side effects. By using a multimodal approach, palliative care healthcare professionals can reduce the dose of medication needed to relieve pain, thereby minimising side effects.
- **Non-pharmacological approaches:** Multimodal approaches often include non-pharmacological therapies such as physiotherapy, acupuncture, massage and relaxation techniques. These approaches complement traditional analgesics and can improve pain management.
- **Psychological support:** Pain at the end of life can be exacerbated by emotional and psychological factors. Multimodal approaches incorporate psychological support strategies to help patients cope with their emotions and reduce their perception of pain.
- **Managing side-effects:** Some pharmacological treatments can cause side-effects that affect the patient's quality of life. Multimodal approaches include interventions to manage these side effects, ensuring that patients benefit from pain relief without adversely affecting other aspects of their health.
- **Interdisciplinary collaboration:** Multimodal approaches often require the collaboration of an interdisciplinary team of healthcare professionals. Doctors, nurses, physical therapists and other specialists work together to create a comprehensive treatment plan.

The use of multimodal approaches to pain management in palliative care makes it possible to offer more complete and effective relief to patients at the end of life. By combining various treatments, these approaches take into account the complexity of pain and help to improve patients' quality of life and comfort while minimising undesirable side effects.

Sensitive and Empathic Communication

The importance of Active Listening and Open Communication

Active listening and open communication are fundamental skills in palliative care, as they create an environment of trust and understanding between healthcare professionals, patients and their families. These elements play a crucial role in providing quality care and addressing the emotional and psychological needs of patients at the end of life.

- **Establishing a bond of trust:** Active listening and open communication help to establish a bond of trust between healthcare professionals and patients. Patients are more inclined to share their concerns, fears and needs when the healthcare professional demonstrates attentive listening.
- **Understanding Needs:** Active listening involves not only hearing the patient's words, but also understanding the emotional message behind those words. This enables palliative care healthcare professionals to better understand the patient's needs and expectations.
- **Acknowledging emotions:** Patients at the end of life can experience a range of complex emotions. Open communication allows patients to express their emotions, while active listening helps healthcare professionals respond with empathy and sensitivity.
- **Informed Decision Making**: Active listening and open communication provide patients and their families with the information they need to make informed decisions about their treatment and care. Patients are better able to make choices that are aligned with their values and preferences.
- **Emotional Support:** Patients at the end of life need emotional support. Active listening and open communication enable healthcare professionals to provide empathetic and compassionate support, helping patients to cope with their emotions.
- **Active participation:** Patients should feel involved in their care. Active listening and open communication promote active participation, encouraging patients to ask questions, express their concerns and make decisions about their care.
- **Reduced anxiety:** When patients feel listened to and understood, their anxiety can be reduced. Open

33

communication reassures patients and their families, helping them to better understand what is happening and to feel in control.

- **Dialogue with Families:** Families often play a crucial role in palliative care. Active listening and open communication include families in the dialogue, allowing them to share their concerns and participate in decision-making.

Active listening and open communication are essential skills that humanise palliative care. They create a respectful and warm environment where patients and their families can express themselves freely and where healthcare professionals can provide care that is adapted, empathetic and centred on the patient's needs.

Tackling the Patient's Difficult Questions and Concerns

Dealing with difficult issues and patient concerns in palliative care requires sensitive, empathetic and respectful communication. Patients at the end of life may have complex and emotional concerns, and palliative care health professionals must be prepared to address these in a way that offers appropriate support.

- **Creating a Safe Space:** Before tackling difficult issues, it is important to create a space where the patient feels comfortable to talk openly. This involves establishing a relationship of trust and listening attentively.
- **Use Accessible Language:** Health professionals in palliative care should use simple, understandable language to explain medical concepts and treatment options. This allows patients to fully understand their situation and the choices available to them.
- **Ask open-ended questions:** Open-ended questions encourage patients to share their thoughts and emotions. Instead of asking questions that require a simple "yes" or "no" answer, healthcare professionals can ask for details and explanations to better understand the patient's concerns.
- **Active listening:** When patients express their concerns, active listening is essential. This means not only hearing the patient's words, but also understanding the emotional context and nuances behind them.
- **Empathy and Validation:** Patients' concerns need to be validated and recognised. Healthcare professionals can

express empathy by acknowledging patients' emotions and showing that they understand the challenges they face.

- **Answer honestly:** Honesty is essential when dealing with difficult issues. Healthcare professionals must provide accurate and transparent information while remaining compassionate and sensitive.
- **Offer options:** When difficult issues are being discussed, it can be helpful to offer options and discuss the pros and cons of each choice. This allows the patient to make informed decisions.
- **Following the patient's lead:** Sometimes patients may not be ready to address certain issues immediately. Palliative care healthcare professionals need to follow the patient's lead and be ready to address concerns when the patient feels ready.
- **Emotional support:** Talking about difficult issues can trigger strong emotions. Healthcare professionals should provide emotional support by offering a sympathetic ear and referring the patient to additional support resources if necessary.
- **Respecting beliefs and values:** When difficult questions arise about a patient's religious, cultural or personal beliefs, it is important to respect them and take them into account in the discussion.

Dealing with difficult issues and patient concerns requires a sensitive and individualised approach. By using effective communication skills and offering emotional support, palliative care healthcare professionals can help patients express their concerns, make informed decisions and feel supported throughout their end-of-life journey.

Creating space for patients' emotional expressions

Palliative care patients can experience a complex range of emotions as they face the end of their lives. Creating a safe and open space for patients to express their emotions is an essential component of palliative care. This enables patients to find emotional support, manage their emotions and maintain their psychological well-being.

- **Empathetic listening:** Healthcare professionals in palliative care must offer empathetic listening to patients who wish to express their emotions. This means being mentally and emotionally present, showing that you understand and care about how they are feeling.

- **Non-judgement:** When patients express their emotions, it is important to create a non-judgmental environment. Patients need to feel safe to share their feelings, even if they are complex or contradictory.
- **Validation of Emotions :** Patients' emotions need to be validated. Healthcare professionals can express their understanding by saying things like "I understand this must be very difficult for you" or "It's normal to feel the way you do".
- **Use encouragement:** Actively encourage patients to express how they are feeling. Ask open-ended questions such as "How do you feel about all this?" or "Are there any specific emotions you'd like to share?"
- **Accepting silence:** Sometimes patients may feel the need to remain silent for a while. Respect these moments of silence and don't feel obliged to fill them with words.
- **Respecting Patient Choice:** Some patients may prefer not to share their emotions verbally. Respect their choices by encouraging them to express their feelings in the way that suits them best, whether that be through art, writing or other forms of expression.
- **Avoiding Immediate Solutions:** When patients express emotions, it is not always necessary to immediately propose solutions. Sometimes it's enough to listen and support them in their feelings.
- **Practise patience:** Some patients may find it difficult to express their emotions because of fear, confusion or sadness. Practise patience and give them time to find the words to express their feelings.
- **Referring to Resources:** If the patient's emotions seem overwhelming, palliative care health professionals can refer patients to additional support resources, such as counsellors, therapists or support groups.

Creating space for patients' emotional expressions is a key element of patient-centred palliative care. It allows patients to find emotional support and to feel heard and understood. By offering a compassionate presence and encouraging open communication, palliative care healthcare professionals contribute to the emotional and psychological well-being of patients at the end of life.

Respect for patient dignity and autonomy

Informed Consent and Active Patient Participation

Informed consent and active patient participation are essential principles in palliative care. They ensure that patients are fully informed about their medical situation, treatment options and rights, and that they play an active role in decision-making about their care at the end of life.

- **Complete information:** Informed consent begins with the provision of complete and comprehensible information about the disease, possible treatments, associated benefits and risks, and potential consequences. This enables the patient to make informed decisions.
- **Accessible language:** Health professionals in palliative care must use clear and accessible language to explain medical concepts. Patients must be able to understand the information and options presented to them.
- **Respect for patients' decisions:** Patients have the right to refuse or choose certain treatments. Healthcare professionals must respect patients' decisions, even if they differ from their recommendations, as long as these decisions are made in full knowledge of the facts.
- **Patient involvement :** Active patient participation means involving patients in the decision-making process. Patients should be encouraged to ask questions, express their concerns and share their preferences.
- **Discussion of Goals:** Palliative care health professionals should discuss with patients their goals of care. This may include prioritising comfort, quality of life and treatment choices according to the patient's preferences.
- **Progressive decisions:** Some decisions in palliative care may be progressive, requiring adjustments as the illness progresses. Patients should be informed of the possibility of reviewing their decisions over time.
- **Respect for Values and Beliefs:** Patient decisions must take account of their values, beliefs and personal

preferences. Healthcare professionals must be sensitive to patients' cultural and religious diversity.

- **Informed   Consent:** Informed consent requires that the patient understands the information provided and then makes a fully informed decision. This may require time and several discussions to clarify points and answer questions.
- **Documentation:** Decisions taken in collaboration with the patient must be accurately documented in the medical record. This ensures that decisions are respected and communicated to members of the care team.
- **Family support:** Involving the family in the decision-making process can be important, particularly when the patient has difficulty communicating or fully understanding information.

Informed consent and active patient participation are fundamental aspects of patient-centred palliative care. They ensure that patients are respected as partners in their own care, promote shared decision-making and enable patients to live their end of life in accordance with their wishes and values.

Respecting patients' end-of-life choices

Respect for patients' end-of-life choices is at the heart of the palliative care philosophy. Patients at the end of life have the right to make informed decisions about how they wish to be treated and cared for as they approach the end of their lives. Respecting these choices ensures that patients maintain their dignity, autonomy and control over their care.

- **Advance   Care Planning:** Advance care planning allows patients to think about and document their end-of-life preferences in advance. This may include decisions about resuscitation, artificial nutrition and hydration, palliative care and other medical treatments.
- **Advance   directives :** Advance directives are written documents that express a patient's wishes regarding end-of-life care. Palliative care professionals must respect these directives and use them to guide treatment decisions.
- **Choice of Place of Death:** Patients have the right to choose where they wish to spend their last moments, whether at home, in a hospice or in hospital. Healthcare

professionals should work to accommodate these preferences as far as possible.

- **Pain relief:** If a patient expresses the wish not to receive aggressive treatments at the end of life, palliative care healthcare professionals must focus on relieving pain and suffering, respecting the patient's choices.
- **Dignity and Comfort:** Respect for the patient's end-of-life choices ensures that care is focused on maintaining dignity, comfort and quality of life. This may include symptom management, the presence of family and friends, and compassionate care.
- **Communication and Listening:** Palliative care health professionals must communicate openly with patients about their end-of-life wishes and preferences. They should also listen carefully to ensure that they understand the patient's choices.
- **Family support:** A patient's end-of-life choices can also have an impact on their family and loved ones. Healthcare professionals must offer emotional and educational support to the family to help them understand and respect the patient's decisions.
- **Ongoing reassessment:** End-of-life choices may evolve as the patient's situation changes. Palliative care professionals must regularly reassess the patient's choices and adapt accordingly.
- **Integration of Culture and Religion:** Cultural and religious beliefs can influence a patient's end-of-life choices. Healthcare professionals must respect and take these aspects into account when making decisions.

Respecting patients' end-of-life choices ensures that their dignity, wishes and values are at the centre of their care. Palliative care healthcare professionals play a crucial role in ensuring that patients can make informed decisions and that these decisions are respected with sensitivity and respect.

Preventing intrusion into patients' privacy and values
In palliative care, respect for the patient's privacy, values and dignity is of paramount importance. Healthcare professionals must be aware of the sensitivity of the situation and endeavour to prevent any unwanted intrusion into the privacy and values of the patient at the end of life.

- **Respectful communication:** Healthcare professionals working in palliative care must adopt a respectful and sensitive approach to communication with patients and their families. This means listening actively, asking questions sensitively and avoiding intrusive communication.
- **Limits to Information Sharing :** Patient medical and personal information should only be shared with those members of the healthcare team who need it to manage the patient. Healthcare professionals must avoid disclosing information without consent.
- **Confidentiality of conversations:** Discussions about illness, treatment and end-of-life choices should take place in private spaces where patients and their families feel comfortable expressing themselves in complete confidence.
- **Consent for Visits:** Visits from healthcare professionals, family members or friends must be coordinated according to the patient's preferences. Healthcare professionals must obtain the patient's consent before allowing access to his or her room.
- **Respect for rituals and beliefs:** Patients may have religious, cultural or personal rituals that are important to them at the end of life. Healthcare professionals must respect these practices and refrain from intervening in an unsolicited manner.
- **Respecting Limits:** Patients may have physical, emotional or psychological limits about what they are willing to share or discuss. Healthcare professionals must respect these limits and not insist on information.
- **Use of Technology :** Communication technologies, such as mobile devices, must be used with discretion and respect. Healthcare professionals must ask permission before taking photographs or recording conversations.
- **Inclusiveness:** Healthcare professionals must be aware of the diversity of cultural and religious values and beliefs. They must avoid imposing their own beliefs and respect those of the patient.
- **Debriefings and Assessments:** The palliative care team can organise regular debriefings to discuss sensitive situations and interactions with patients. This allows approaches to be adjusted to prevent intrusion into the patient's privacy and values.

Respect for the patient's privacy and values is an essential element of patient-centred palliative care. Palliative care healthcare professionals play a crucial role in creating an environment where patients feel respected, listened to and in control of their own choices and privacy at the end of life.

Chapter 3:
Assessment and Planning Palliative Care

Initial Assessment of the Patient in Palliative Care

Complete Collection of Medical and Social History

Gathering a complete medical and social history of the palliative care patient is a fundamental step in ensuring high-quality, personalised care. This involves gathering not only medical information, but also details about the patient's life, preferences, relationships and specific needs. A well-understood medical and social history enables palliative care healthcare professionals to better understand the patient as a whole and to provide care that meets their physical, psychological and social needs.

- **Medical history:** Collecting a patient's medical history includes information on past illnesses, current diagnoses, previous treatments, allergies and the results of medical examinations. This helps to understand the patient's medical history.
- **Evolution of the disease:** Understanding how the disease has evolved over time is crucial to identifying the patient's current needs and planning future care. This includes key milestones, symptoms experienced and previous treatments.
- **Ongoing treatments:** Current medical treatments, such as drugs, therapies and interventions, must be accurately documented to ensure continuity and to adjust palliative care accordingly.
- **Treatment preferences:** Understanding patients' treatment preferences, including limitations and priorities, helps to ensure that palliative care is aligned with their wishes.
- **Social History:** Gathering information about the patient's social life, such as family, friends, interests, values and activities, helps to understand what is important to them and to create a person-centred approach to care.

- **Support network:** Identifying members of the patient's support network, such as family, friends and relatives, enables healthcare professionals to work with them to provide holistic care.
- **Living situation:** Understanding where the patient lives, what their living conditions are and whether they need home assistance or other adjustments to their environment is crucial to ensuring their comfort and safety.
- **Psychological needs:** Gathering information about the patient's emotional needs, concerns, anxieties and psychological goals enables healthcare professionals to provide appropriate support.
- **Cultural and Religious Preferences:** Knowing the patient's cultural and religious preferences means that care and communication can be adapted to respect their beliefs and practices.
- **Previous care plans:** Examining the patient's previous care plans and medical choices helps us to better understand their care trajectory and to adapt to changes.

Gathering a complete medical and social history of the palliative care patient ensures that care is individualised and focused on the needs of the whole patient. This enables palliative care healthcare professionals to design tailored care plans and provide holistic support throughout the patient's end-of-life journey.

Assessment of Current Quality of Life and Symptoms

Assessing current quality of life and symptoms is a central part of palliative care. This stage enables healthcare professionals to gain an in-depth understanding of the patient's situation, suffering and needs, so that they can put in place targeted interventions to improve quality of life.

- **Quality of Life Assessment:** Quality of life for patients at the end of life is not just about managing physical symptoms. It also encompasses emotional, social and psychological aspects. Healthcare professionals need to discuss the patient's preferences, expectations and quality of life goals.
- **Assessment of Physical Symptoms:** Healthcare professionals need to accurately assess the patient's

physical symptoms, such as pain, nausea, fatigue, dyspnoea and other symptoms associated with their medical condition. This allows effective treatments to be prescribed to relieve suffering.

- **Use of Rating Scales:** Rating scales for pain, fatigue, depression and other symptoms are important tools for quantifying the intensity of symptoms and monitoring changes over time. This allows decisions to be made based on objective data.
- **Assessment of Emotional Symptoms:** Emotional symptoms, such as anxiety, depression, fear and psychological distress, must also be assessed. Healthcare professionals must take into account the psychological impact of the illness and the end-of-life process on the patient.
- **Assessment of Social Symptoms: The** patient's social problems and needs must be taken into account, such as family relationships, social support, isolation and financial concerns.
- **Regular interviews:** The assessment of symptoms and quality of life must be continuous and regular, as the patient's situation can change rapidly. The interviews enable care to be adjusted to meet changing needs.
- **Treatment objectives :** The patient's treatment goals should be aligned with managing their symptoms and improving their quality of life. Healthcare professionals should discuss treatment options and their associated pros and cons with the patient.
- **Holistic approach:** Symptoms and quality of life should be assessed from a holistic perspective, taking into account the many facets of the patient's well-being.
- **Patient involvement:** Healthcare professionals must actively involve patients in the assessment of their symptoms and quality of life. Open communication and shared decision-making strengthen patient-healthcare professional collaboration.

Assessing current quality of life and symptoms is a key element of palliative care. It guides treatment decisions, relieves suffering and improves quality of life for patients at the end of life. By tailoring care to the patient's individual needs, palliative care healthcare professionals promote a holistic and personalised approach.

Identification of Patient Care Preferences and Objectives

Identifying the patient's preferences and goals of care is a crucial step in palliative care. This involves working collaboratively with the patient to understand their wishes, needs and priorities at the end of life. This helps to personalise care, make informed treatment decisions and ensure that the patient's choices are respected.

- **Open discussions:** Palliative care health professionals should engage in open and honest discussions with the patient to discover their preferences and goals. This may include conversations about priorities, acceptable treatments and treatment limits.
- **Treatment preferences: It is** essential to understand the patient's treatment preferences, such as the medical options they wish to pursue or avoid. These preferences guide treatment decisions while respecting the patient's values.
- **Quality of life:** Healthcare professionals should discuss the patient's vision of quality of life. This enables them to define care objectives aimed at improving or maintaining their quality of life in line with their priorities.
- **Treatment limits:** Identifying treatment limits is crucial to avoid any undesirable or unnecessary medical intervention. Patients can express their limits in terms of resuscitation, artificial ventilation, artificial feeding, etc.
- **Comfort Goals:** Patient care goals may focus on pain relief, symptom management and comfort rather than aggressive healing. Healthcare professionals need to adapt care accordingly.
- **Preferences for Place of Death:** Patients often have preferences about where they wish to spend their final moments. These preferences must be respected and taken into account when planning care.
- **Ongoing communication:** Preferences and goals of care can change over time. Healthcare professionals need to maintain ongoing communication to ensure that care remains aligned with the patient's wishes.
- **Family Involvement:** Involving the patient's family in discussions about preferences and goals of care can help ensure that decisions are well understood and supported.

- **Documenting decisions: The** patient's preferences and goals of care must be clearly documented in their medical record. This ensures that the patient's choices are respected by the entire care team.

Identifying the patient's preferences and goals of care promotes a person-centred approach to care at the end of life. By honouring the patient's choices and engaging in open communication, palliative care healthcare professionals ensure that care is aligned with the patient's individual needs, values and wishes.

Drawing up a Personalised Care Plan

Integration of Patient Needs and Concerns
Integrating the patient's needs and concerns is an essential component of palliative care. It involves gathering information from the patient and their family, and then designing a comprehensive care plan that addresses their physical, emotional, social and spiritual needs. Successful integration of these needs ensures that care is personalised and patient-centred at the end of life.

- **Holistic approach: The** needs of the patient at the end of life are not limited to their physical symptoms. Palliative care professionals must take a holistic approach that considers all aspects of the patient's life, including emotions, relationships, values and concerns.
- **Personalised Care Plan:** Using the information gathered during the assessment, palliative care health professionals should work with the patient to develop a personalised care plan. This plan should reflect the patient's treatment goals, preferences and priorities.
- **Relieving Suffering:** The need to relieve pain and suffering is at the heart of palliative care. The care plan should include strategies to effectively manage physical and emotional symptoms.
- **Symptom Management:** Based on symptom assessment, the care plan should include specific approaches to managing each symptom, using pharmacological and non-pharmacological treatments.

- **Psychological support:** If the patient expresses emotional and psychological needs, the care plan should include interventions to provide appropriate support, such as supportive therapy, mediation and counselling.
- **Taking preferences into account:** The care plan must reflect the patient's preferences and choices regarding treatment, including treatment limits and quality of life objectives.
- **Communication:** The care plan should include guidelines for maintaining open and regular communication between the patient, their family and the care team. This ensures that needs continue to be addressed over time.
- **Family Support:** The needs and concerns of the patient's family must also be taken into account in the care plan. This may include emotional support, information about care and end-of-life planning.
- **Ongoing adaptation:** The care plan must be flexible and able to adapt to changes in the patient's condition and changing needs. Regular adjustments must be made as the situation evolves.

Successfully integrating the patient's needs and concerns into the care plan ensures a personalised and respectful approach at the end of life. By placing the patient at the centre of decision-making and addressing his or her needs as a whole, palliative care healthcare professionals promote a comfortable, dignified and person-centred end-of-life experience.

Interdisciplinary Collaboration for Planning
Interdisciplinary collaboration plays an essential role in palliative care planning. Comprehensive and holistic care of the patient at the end of life requires a team of healthcare professionals working together to meet their complex needs. Interdisciplinary collaboration ensures that care is well coordinated, comprehensive and patient-centred.

- **Palliative Care Team:** The palliative care team is made up of healthcare professionals from different disciplines, such as doctors, nurses, social workers, psychologists, spiritual advisors and other experts. Each brings their own expertise to provide comprehensive care.

47

- **Team meetings:** The professionals on the palliative care team should meet regularly to discuss the patient's situation, share information, assess needs and adjust the care plan accordingly.
- **Information Sharing:** Team members need to share relevant patient information effectively, including assessment results, goals of care, preferences and limitations. This ensures coordinated care.
- **Collaborative planning:** Care planning should be collaborative, involving all members of the interdisciplinary team. Each member contributes their expertise to create an overall care plan.
- **Role Assignment:** Each professional in the palliative care team should have clear roles and responsibilities in implementing the care plan. This avoids duplication and ensures an organised approach.
- **Transparent communication:** Transparent communication between team members is essential to avoid misunderstandings and ensure smooth patient care.
- **Ongoing training:** Team members need to keep abreast of the latest developments in their respective fields in order to offer the most up-to-date care and best practice.
- **Meeting multiple needs:** Palliative care patients often have complex needs that encompass medical, emotional, psychological and spiritual aspects. Interdisciplinary collaboration makes it possible to meet all these needs.
- **Shared Decision Making:** Members of the palliative care team must work closely with the patient and family to make informed treatment decisions that respect the patient's choices.
- **Flexibility and adaptability:** A patient's situation can change rapidly at the end of life. The palliative care team must be ready to adjust the care plan to meet changing needs.

Interdisciplinary collaboration is the cornerstone of quality palliative care. By working together, healthcare professionals can offer coherent, comprehensive and holistic care that improves the quality of life of patients at the end of life and supports their dignity and well-being.

Short- and long-term planning
Short-term and long-term planning is an essential approach in palliative care. It aims to anticipate the patient's needs both in the short term, to manage current symptoms and problems, and in the long term, to foresee possible developments and necessary adjustments. This proactive approach ensures continuity of care and holistic management throughout the patient's trajectory at the end of life.

Short-term planning :
- **Symptom Management:** Short-term planning focuses on the effective management of the patient's current symptoms. Healthcare professionals work to relieve pain, dyspnoea, nausea and other uncomfortable symptoms.
- **Rapid response: The** patient's urgent needs are identified and dealt with quickly. This may include medication adjustments, medical interventions or strategies to improve comfort.
- **Emotional support: In the** event of acute emotional or psychological distress, supportive interventions are put in place to help patients cope with their emotions.
- **Regular communication:** Regular communication between the patient, their family and the care team enables progress to be monitored, care to be adjusted as the situation evolves and immediate concerns to be addressed.

Long-term planning :
- **Predicting the future:** Palliative care healthcare professionals work with the patient and their family to envisage possible developments in their medical condition. This helps to anticipate future needs.
- **End-of-life planning:** If the patient expresses a wish to plan the practical aspects of their end of life, such as comfort care, death location and funeral arrangements, these are discussed and documented.
- **Managing change:** A patient's situation can change rapidly. Long-term planning takes these changes into account and provides for possible adjustments in the care plan.
- **Evolving Care Plan:** The long-term care plan is evolving and flexible to meet new needs as they arise over time.

- **Advance directive:** If the patient expresses specific wishes regarding end-of-life treatment, such as refusing cardiopulmonary resuscitation, these wishes are respected and documented.
- **Ongoing support:** Healthcare professionals offer ongoing support to patients and their families, providing information and answering questions about the various stages at the end of life.

Short- and long-term planning ensures that palliative care is adapted to the changing needs of the patient at the end of life. By taking into account both current problems and future challenges, palliative care healthcare professionals ensure comprehensive, proactive and patient-centred care.

Symptom and Medical Problem Management

Pharmacological and Non-pharmacological Approaches to Symptoms

Managing symptoms in palliative care requires a multidimensional approach that combines both pharmacological and non-pharmacological interventions. This holistic approach aims to relieve the suffering of patients at the end of life using a variety of approaches tailored to their specific needs.

Pharmacological approaches :
- **Pain management:** Analgesics, such as opioids and non-steroidal anti-inflammatory drugs, are commonly used to relieve pain. Titration is essential to adjust doses and optimise relief while minimising side effects.
- **Control of Respiratory Symptoms:** For dyspnoea (difficulty breathing), bronchodilators, opioids and other drugs may be prescribed to improve the patient's breathing.
- **Management of Nausea and Vomiting:** Antiemetics are used to control nausea and vomiting. The choice of medication depends on the underlying cause and patient preference.
- **Anxiety relief:** Benzodiazepines can be prescribed to relieve anxiety and agitation in patients. However, their use must be cautious to avoid excessive sedation.

50

- **Treatment of depression:** Antidepressants may be recommended to treat the depression that can occur at the end of life. The choice of medication will depend on the patient's situation.

Non-pharmacological approaches :

- **Complementary therapies:** Approaches such as acupuncture, massage therapy, reflexology and music therapy can offer symptomatic relief as a complement to pharmacological treatments.
- **Supportive Therapy:** Psychotherapy, group therapy and family therapy can help patients cope with their emotions, reduce anxiety and improve their psychological well-being.
- **Physical therapies:** Physiotherapy can help maintain mobility and prevent complications associated with immobility.
- **Comfort Palliative Care:** Comfort palliative care includes interventions to improve physical comfort, such as repositioning, temperature management and oral hygiene.
- **Spiritual support:** Spiritual and religious advisers can offer emotional and spiritual support to patients at the end of life, helping them to find meaning and peace at this time.
- **Art therapies:** Art therapy, dance therapy and other forms of creative therapy can help patients to express their emotions and find a way to express themselves at the end of life.

The combined approach of pharmacological and non-pharmacological approaches enables palliative care healthcare professionals to respond effectively to the complex needs of patients at the end of life. By adapting interventions to the patient's individual situation, we promote overall relief of suffering and improved quality of life.

Managing Emotional and Psychological Symptoms

Managing emotional and psychological symptoms is a crucial part of palliative care, as patients at the end of life often experience a complex range of emotions and psychological suffering. Managing these symptoms aims to improve the patient's emotional well-being, promote a healthy grieving process and provide support for a peaceful transition to the end of life.

Psychological and Emotional Approaches :
- **Psychological support:** Palliative care healthcare professionals, including psychologists and counsellors, offer emotional support by providing spaces for discussing fears, worries and feelings related to the end of life.
- **Supportive therapy:** Psychotherapy, particularly cognitive behavioural therapy (CBT), can help treat depression, anxiety and other common emotional disorders.
- **Anxiety Management:** Relaxation techniques, deep breathing, meditation and mindfulness are used to help reduce anxiety and promote a sense of calm.
- **Emotional expression:** Encouraging patients to express their emotions can help relieve emotional tension. Art therapy, writing and other forms of creative expression can be used to this end.
- **Anticipatory Bereavement Management:** Patients at the end of life may experience anticipatory bereavement for their own lives. Discussions on this subject, together with advice and resources on bereavement, can help to facilitate this process.
- **Spiritual support:** Spiritual or religious counsellors can help patients address spiritual issues and find comfort in their faith during this time.

Pharmacotherapeutic approaches :
- **Antidepressants:** If depression is present, antidepressants can be prescribed to help reduce depressive symptoms and improve emotional well-being.
- **Anxiolytics:** Anxiolytics can be used to reduce anxiety and agitation in patients at the end of life, but should be used with caution to avoid excessive sedation.
- **Mild sedation:** In some cases, mild sedation may be used to relieve agitation and severe emotional discomfort in terminally ill patients.
- **Symptom control:** By improving the management of physical symptoms, such as pain and dyspnoea, healthcare professionals often help to reduce the associated emotional symptoms.
- **Family Education and Support:** Families should be made aware of the emotional symptoms the patient may be experiencing and encouraged to provide support and reassurance.

Managing emotional and psychological symptoms in palliative care helps to improve a patient's quality of life at the end of life and promotes a peaceful transition process. Using a combination of therapeutic and supportive approaches, healthcare professionals help patients cope with their emotions and find meaning and comfort during this delicate period.

Adaptation of the Care Plan according to changes in the patient's condition

Adapting the care plan to the patient's changing condition is a crucial aspect of palliative care. Patients at the end of life can experience rapid and unpredictable changes in their medical condition, and it is essential that healthcare professionals are prepared to adjust care to meet changing needs. This adaptation ensures that patients receive appropriate and personalised care throughout their end-of-life trajectory.

- **Ongoing monitoring:** Healthcare professionals must regularly monitor the condition of the patient at the end of life. This may include checking vital signs, assessing symptoms and observing changes in their overall condition.
- **Regular assessment**: Regular assessments of the patient's condition help to detect any new symptoms or changes in their medical condition at an early stage. This information guides the necessary adjustments in the care plan.
- **Open communication:** Communication between the patient, their family and the care team is essential to share information about changes and new needs. This enables informed decision-making.
- **Flexibility in treatment:** Pharmacological and non-pharmacological treatments must be flexible and adapted to the patient's current symptoms and needs.
- **Readjustment of Objectives:** If the patient's condition deteriorates, the objectives of care may evolve from symptom management to support more focused on comfort and quality of life.
- **Emotional   support:** Changes in a patient's condition can have an emotional impact on them and their family. Psychological and emotional support interventions must be adapted accordingly.

- **Evolving   Care Plan:** The care plan should be seen as a living document, capable of adjusting to the patient's changing needs.
- **Transition planning:** If the patient's condition indicates an imminent transition to the end of life, discussions on end-of-life planning and comfort care should be initiated.
- **Honest   conversations:** If the patient's condition is declining, healthcare professionals need to have open and honest conversations with the patient and family to explain changes and care options.
- **Respect for Patient Choice:** Even when a patient's condition deteriorates, their treatment choices and wishes should be respected and followed as far as possible.

Continuously adapting the care plan as the patient's condition changes ensures that palliative care remains appropriate and patient-centred. By being attentive to changing needs and adjusting interventions accordingly, palliative care healthcare professionals provide comprehensive and responsive support to ensure the patient's comfort, dignity and quality of life at the end of life.

Chapter 4:
Pain Management and Symptoms

Pain Assessment and Use of Rating Scales

Differentiation between Acute and Chronic Pain
The distinction between acute and chronic pain is essential in palliative care, as it guides pain management approaches and treatment choices for patients at the end of life. Understanding the differences between these two types of pain enables healthcare professionals to provide appropriate and effective relief, while improving the patient's quality of life.

Acute pain :
- **Underlying Cause:** Acute pain is usually caused by an identifiable injury, illness or trauma. It is often the result of tissue damage, inflammation or a medical procedure.
- **Sudden onset:** Acute pain usually begins suddenly and can be intense. It is often associated with an acute medical condition or procedure.
- **Limited duration:** Acute pain is usually short-lived, lasting from a few hours to a few weeks, and diminishes as the underlying cause is treated or healed.
- **Predictability:** Acute pain is often predictable in terms of cause and duration. It diminishes as the healing process progresses.
- **Response to Treatment:** Acute pain generally responds well to medical treatments, such as analgesics, and management of the underlying cause.

Chronic pain :
- **Underlying cause :** Chronic pain can be caused by chronic diseases, nerve damage, inflammatory conditions or other complex factors. The cause can be difficult to identify.
- **Prolonged duration:** Chronic pain generally lasts for more than three months, or even indefinitely. It can persist even after the initial cause has healed.

- **Variable intensity:** Chronic pain can vary in intensity over time, from mild to severe. It may have periods of temporary relief followed by relapses.
- **Influence on Quality of Life:** Chronic pain can have a significant impact on a patient's quality of life, affecting sleep, mood, mobility and daily activities.
- **Response to Treatment :** Chronic pain can be more difficult to manage and may not respond as effectively to conventional treatments. A multidisciplinary approach is often required.

By understanding the difference between acute and chronic pain, palliative care healthcare professionals can tailor their pain management strategies to the specific needs of the patient. They can provide targeted care aimed at reducing pain and improving quality of life, taking into account the physical, emotional and psychological aspects of the patient's suffering at the end of life.

Pain Assessment Methods: Visual Scales, Numerical Scales, etc.

Accurate pain assessment is fundamental to effective pain management in palliative care. Healthcare professionals use different assessment methods to understand the intensity and characteristics of the pain experienced by the patient. These assessments provide essential information for adapting treatments and interventions, thereby ensuring optimal pain relief.

Visual Analogue Scale (VAS): The VAS is a graphic scale on which patients mark their pain on a straight line, ranging from no pain (0) to the maximum pain imaginable (10). This method provides a simple, visual way of measuring pain intensity.

Numerical scale (EN): The EN is a scale in which the patient assigns a number to their pain, usually from 0 to 10, to indicate its intensity. It is similar to the VAS but does not include the visual aspect.

Simple Verbal Scale (EVS): The EVS asks the patient to choose one of several terms (such as "no pain", "mild pain", "moderate pain", "severe pain", etc.) to describe their level of pain.

Digital Verbal Scale (DVS): The VNS combines elements of the verbal and numerical scales. The patient chooses an adjective from a list (such as "no pain", "mild pain", "moderate pain", "severe pain") and then assigns a number to indicate the intensity of the pain.

Self-assessment questionnaires: Some questionnaires, such as the McGill Pain Index (MDI), allow patients to describe their pain using specific words and phrases to describe the characteristics of their pain, such as its quality and location.

Continuous assessment: In palliative care, pain assessment must be continuous and regular, as the intensity and characteristics of pain can change. Patients should be encouraged to express their pain at any time.

Holistic approach: In addition to assessment scales, palliative care healthcare professionals also consider the patient's verbal and non-verbal expressions, as well as psychological, emotional and contextual factors that may influence the perception of pain. The use of different pain assessment methods enables palliative care healthcare professionals to gather comprehensive information on the intensity and characteristics of the pain experienced by the patient. This ensures that pain treatments are precisely tailored and that pain relief is optimal, helping to improve the patient's quality of life at the end of life.

The Importance of Communication with the Patient for Accurate Assessment

Open and effective communication between the patient and the care team is crucial for accurate pain assessment in palliative care. Patients at the end of life may experience a range of emotions, fears and concerns related to their pain, and careful communication allows healthcare professionals to fully understand their experience, leading to better pain management.

Accurate expression of pain: Patients are the most reliable source of information about their own pain. By encouraging open communication, patients can describe the nature, intensity, location and characteristics of their pain, which helps healthcare professionals to assess the situation more accurately.

Influence of Emotions: Pain at the end of life can be influenced by emotional factors such as anxiety, fear, sadness and frustration. Patients can describe how their emotions interact with their pain, allowing for a more holistic approach to management.

Evolution of Pain: Patients can explain how their pain evolves over time. This includes the times when the pain is most intense, the times when it is relieved and the factors that seem to influence these variations.

Response to Treatments: Open communication allows patients to describe how they respond to pain treatments, which guides necessary adjustments and helps avoid unwanted side effects.

Treatment preferences : Patients can express their treatment preferences, including their previous experiences with certain drugs or approaches, enabling healthcare professionals to tailor treatment options.

Impact on Quality of Life: Patients can explain how their pain affects their overall quality of life, including their ability to sleep, interact socially, move around and participate in meaningful activities.

Trust and Empowerment: Open communication builds trust between the patient and the care team, which can lead to the patient feeling more involved in decisions about their own pain management.

Taking cultural factors into account: Careful communication also allows patients to share cultural or spiritual factors that may influence their perception of pain and their treatment preferences.

Communication with the patient is a cornerstone of accurate pain assessment in palliative care. By establishing a space of trust where patients can express their sensations, needs and concerns, healthcare professionals can better understand pain in the overall context of the patient's life, leading to more effective and empathetic pain management.

Pharmacological and non-pharmacological approaches

Analgesics: Assessment and Appropriate Administration
Analgesics play a central role in pain management in palliative care. Careful assessment of the patient's pain and individual needs is essential to determine the appropriate choice of analgesics and their administration. The aim is to provide optimal relief while minimising undesirable side effects.

Pain Assessment: Before prescribing an analgesic, healthcare professionals must carry out a full assessment of the patient's pain. This includes the use of pain scales, discussion with the patient about the intensity, quality and location of the pain, and consideration of emotional and psychological factors.

Choice of analgesic: Depending on the assessment, the healthcare professional will choose an analgesic suited to the intensity and characteristics of the pain. Analgesics are generally classified into three levels: non-opioid analgesics, weak opioids and strong opioids.

Non-opioid analgesics: These are generally used for mild to moderate pain. They include drugs such as paracetamol and non-steroidal anti-inflammatory drugs (NSAIDs). The advantages of these drugs are their generally low side-effect profile.

Weak opioids: For moderate to severe pain, weak opioids such as codeine and tramadol may be prescribed. They have a higher potential for side effects than non-opioid analgesics, but offer more powerful relief.

Strong opioids: Strong opioids, such as morphine, oxycodone and fentanyl, are used for severe and chronic pain. They are effective in relieving intense pain, but require close monitoring because of the increased risk of side effects.

Suitable administration: Analgesics are generally administered orally in the form of tablets, liquids or skin patches. However, in cases where the patient cannot swallow or absorb oral medication, other routes of administration, such as subcutaneous, intramuscular or intravenous injection, may be used.

Titration and equianalgesia: Titration involves adjusting analgesic doses according to the intensity of the patient's pain. Equianalgesia makes it possible to convert doses from one analgesic to another while maintaining equivalent relief.

Side Effects and Management: Healthcare professionals should carefully monitor the side effects of analgesics, such as sedation, constipation, nausea and vomiting. Specific interventions, such as anti-constipation medication, may be required to mitigate these effects.

By tailoring pain assessment and the choice of analgesics to the patient's individual needs, palliative care healthcare professionals aim to provide optimal relief while minimising undesirable side effects. Open communication with the patient is essential to adjust doses according to the evolution of pain and responses to treatment, thus ensuring maximum comfort throughout the end-of-life period.

Use of Relaxation and Meditation Techniques

In palliative care, pain management is not limited to the use of medication. Relaxation and meditation techniques play an important role in holistic pain management. These non-pharmacological approaches offer patients at the end of life tools to manage their pain in a complementary way and enhance their emotional well-being.

Relaxation Techniques :
- **Deep breathing:** Teaching patients deep breathing techniques can help reduce muscle tension and promote relaxation, which can contribute to partial pain relief.
- **Progressive Muscle Relaxation:** This method involves gradually contracting and releasing different muscle groups to induce deep relaxation and reduce tension.
- **Guided imagery:** By guiding patients through positive, soothing visualisations, healthcare professionals can help to divert attention from pain and create a sense of calm.
- **Therapeutic massage:** Gentle massages can reduce muscle tension, promote circulation and induce a feeling of general relaxation, which can help manage pain.

Meditation Techniques :
- **Mindfulness meditation:** By concentrating on the present moment, patients can develop greater tolerance to pain by observing their sensations and thoughts without judgement.
- **Visualisation Meditation:** Patients are guided through positive visualisations to create a peaceful and relaxed state of mind, which can help to reduce the perception of pain.
- **Transcendental Meditation:** This technique involves the silent repetition of a mantra to calm the mind and promote relaxation, which can be useful for relieving pain.
- **Breath Meditation:** By concentrating on breathing, patients can calm their minds and create a mental separation from the pain.

Personalised techniques: Relaxation and meditation techniques should be adapted to the patient's individual preferences and abilities. Some people may prefer silent meditation, while others may find muscle relaxation more effective.

Integration into Holistic Care: Relaxation and meditation techniques do not replace medical treatments, but are often used as a complement to offer a holistic approach to pain management.

Training and Encouragement: Patients can benefit from sessions teaching and practising these techniques, and it is important to encourage them to use them regularly to reap the full benefits.

By integrating relaxation and meditation techniques into palliative care, healthcare professionals are providing patients with practical tools to manage pain proactively. These approaches enable patients to feel more autonomous in their pain relief process, while also strengthening their emotional and mental well-being during this sensitive period.

Integration of Complementary Therapies to Relieve Symptoms

In palliative care, the integration of complementary therapies can play a significant role in relieving the physical, emotional and psychological symptoms of patients at the end of life. These holistic approaches are designed to complement traditional medical treatments and offer a more comprehensive approach to symptom management, thereby improving patients' quality of life.

Symptom Relief Therapies :
- **Massage therapy:** Therapeutic massages can reduce muscle tension, improve blood circulation and reduce physical discomfort.
- **Acupuncture:** Acupuncture can help reduce pain, nausea, vomiting and sleep disorders, while promoting a sense of relaxation.
- **Aromatherapy:** Essential oils can be used to alleviate anxiety, insomnia and other emotional symptoms, as well as to improve physical comfort.
- **Reflexology:** This technique applies pressure to specific points on the feet and hands to promote relaxation and relieve pain.
- **Music therapy:** Listening to soothing music can reduce anxiety, improve mood and create a calm environment.

- **Art therapy:** Drawing, painting and other forms of artistic expression can help patients to express their emotions, relax and find a sense of achievement.

Personalised approach: It is essential to tailor complementary therapies to the patient's individual needs and preferences. What works for one patient may not work for another.

Ongoing assessment: Healthcare professionals should carefully monitor the patient's response to complementary therapies and make adjustments if necessary.

Multidisciplinary Care Team: Complementary therapies should be integrated as part of a comprehensive and co-ordinated approach involving different members of the care team, including doctors, nurses, social workers and specialist therapists.

Scientific validation: Although complementary therapies have shown benefits in relieving symptoms, it is important to choose approaches with a solid scientific basis and to integrate them judiciously.

The integration of complementary therapies into palliative care offers patients additional options for managing their symptoms and improving their overall well-being. By combining these approaches with conventional medical treatments, healthcare professionals can offer a full range of support to patients at the end of life, while respecting their individual preferences and seeking to meet their physical and emotional needs.

Managing Other Common Symptoms

Nausea and Vomiting : Medical and Preventive Treatments

Nausea and vomiting are common symptoms in palliative care, and may be the result of the underlying illness, medical treatments or emotional factors. Effective management of these symptoms is essential to improve the quality of life of patients at the end of life. Approaches include medical treatments and preventive strategies aimed at reducing the incidence and severity of these symptoms.

Medical treatments :
- **Antiemetics:** Antiemetics are medicines designed to prevent or treat nausea and vomiting. They work by blocking the signals in the brain responsible for these symptoms. Different classes of antiemetics can be used

depending on the cause and severity of the nausea and vomiting.

- **Anticholinergic** drugs: These block the signals between nerves and muscles, which can help reduce the stomach contractions responsible for nausea and vomiting.
- **Prokinetic drugs:** Prokinetic drugs help speed up the movement of food through the stomach and intestines, which can reduce feelings of nausea.

Preventive strategies :

- **Pain management:** Untreated pain can aggravate nausea and vomiting. Adequate pain management can therefore help to reduce these symptoms.
- **Hydration:** Keeping the patient well hydrated can help prevent nausea and vomiting. However, frequent small amounts of fluid are often better tolerated than large amounts all at once.
- **Balanced diet:** A balanced, light diet can minimise nausea. Avoiding fatty, spicy and odour-rich foods can help.
- **Avoid strong odours:** Strong odours can trigger nausea. Avoiding environments with strong odours can help prevent symptoms.
- **Stress and anxiety management:** Stress and anxiety can make nausea worse. Relaxation techniques, meditation and other psychological approaches can help.

Personalisation: As every patient is unique, it is important to tailor treatments to individual needs and preferences.

Communication and Ongoing Assessment: Healthcare professionals need to maintain open communication with patients to monitor the effectiveness of treatments and adjust strategies accordingly.

The management of nausea and vomiting in palliative care aims to provide effective relief while minimising undesirable side effects. By combining targeted medical treatments with preventive strategies and taking into account the patient's specific needs, healthcare professionals help to improve the patient's comfort and quality of life during this sensitive period.

Fatigue and Weakness: Approaches to Managing Lassitude

Fatigue and weakness are common symptoms in palliative care patients, and can have a significant impact on quality of life.

Effectively managing lassitude requires a multidisciplinary approach that combines medical, behavioural and psychological strategies to help patients conserve their energy and maintain a degree of comfort.

Medical Strategies :
- **Comprehensive assessment:** A thorough assessment of fatigue is essential to identify underlying causes, whether related to the disease itself, to treatments or to other medical factors.
- **Optimising medication:** Medications that contribute to fatigue can be adjusted or replaced if possible. Managing the side effects of medication can also help reduce fatigue.
- **Managing Related Symptoms:** Symptoms such as pain, nausea, sleep problems and depression can make fatigue worse. By treating these symptoms, fatigue can be better controlled.

Behavioural strategies :
- **Energy management:** Encourage patients to manage their energy wisely by planning activities for the times of day when they feel most energetic. Regular rest periods are also important.
- **Gentle physical activity:** Although rest is important, gentle physical activity, such as walking or yoga, can help maintain muscle strength and improve endurance.
- **Balanced nutrition:** A balanced diet rich in nutrients can help maintain energy. Light, frequent meals may be better tolerated than large ones.

Psychological strategies :
- **Stress management:** Stress and anxiety can contribute to fatigue. Relaxation, meditation and breathing techniques can help manage these factors.
- **Psychological support:** Offering psychological and emotional support to patients can help them cope with fatigue and better understand their associated emotions.
- **Setting Realistic Goals:** Encouraging patients to set realistic goals for the day can avoid activity overload and help prevent increased fatigue.

Ongoing assessment: Healthcare professionals should carefully monitor patient fatigue and adjust strategies accordingly, based on disease progression and response to treatment.

Managing fatigue and weakness in palliative care requires a holistic approach that takes into account medical, behavioural and psychological aspects. By tailoring strategies to the patient's individual needs and working closely with the care team, healthcare professionals aim to improve the patient's quality of life by promoting a better balance between activity and rest.

Dyspnoea (Breathing Difficulty) : Strategies to Improve Breathing

Dyspnoea, or difficulty breathing, is a common symptom in palliative care, often caused by advanced lung disease, heart problems or other medical conditions. Effectively managing dyspnoea is crucial to improving a patient's quality of life and enabling them to breathe more easily. Approaches include medical and behavioural strategies to relieve breathing discomfort.

Medical Strategies :
- **Comprehensive assessment:** A thorough assessment of dyspnoea is essential to identify underlying causes and determine whether they are related to lung, heart or other conditions.
- **Treatment Optimisation:** Existing treatments for underlying medical conditions should be optimised to minimise dyspnoea. This may include adjusting medications and specific interventions.
- **Oxygen therapy:** In some cases, administration of oxygen may be beneficial to improve oxygen intake and relieve dyspnoea.

Behavioural strategies :
- **Positioning:** Encourage patients to adopt positions that facilitate breathing, such as sitting slightly forward or using pillows to elevate the head.
- **Controlled breathing:** Teaching patients slow, deep breathing techniques can help improve breathing efficiency and reduce anxiety linked to dyspnoea.
- **Ventilation:** Using portable ventilators or air vents in the patient's room can promote air circulation and make breathing easier.

Psychological support :
- **Managing anxiety:** Dyspnoea can cause anxiety. By using relaxation techniques, meditation and psychological

support, patients can better manage the anxiety associated with their breathing difficulties.

- **Communication:** Encouraging patients to express their feelings and concerns about dyspnoea can help reduce emotional stress and improve their general well-being.

Ongoing assessment: Healthcare professionals should carefully monitor the patient's dyspnoea and adjust strategies according to disease progression and response to treatment.

Dyspnoea management in palliative care aims to improve patients' quality of life by enabling them to breathe more comfortably. By combining medical and behavioural approaches tailored to the patient's individual needs, healthcare professionals help to relieve respiratory discomfort and help patients to cope better with this difficulty.

Chapter 5:
Psychological and emotional support

The importance of psychological support in palliative care

Recognising the Emotional Impact of Terminal Illness

Terminal illness has a profound and complex impact on patients' emotions and emotional well-being. Recognising this emotional impact is crucial to providing adequate and holistic support to patients at the end of life. Palliative care healthcare professionals must be sensitive to the patient's emotions and be prepared to address these aspects with compassion and empathy.

Variety of Emotions: Terminally ill patients may experience a range of intense emotions, including fear, anxiety, sadness, anger, frustration and sometimes even a sense of relief or acceptance. Each individual reacts differently to the reality of their situation.

Psychological impact: Confronting one's own mortality can lead to a variety of psychological concerns, such as loss of control, feelings of powerlessness, concern for loved ones, regret and existential questions about life and death.

Active listening: Healthcare professionals must offer patients active listening to enable them to express their emotions in complete confidence. It is important to create a safe space where patients can share their thoughts and feelings without judgement.

Validation of emotions: Validation of emotions is essential. Patients need to know that their emotions are normal and understandable in the face of the difficult situation they are facing.

Open Communication: Healthcare professionals should encourage open and honest communication with patients about their emotions. This can help identify sources of emotional distress and develop strategies to deal with them.

Psychological support: Referring patients to psychologists, social workers or mental health counsellors who specialise in palliative care can offer additional emotional support in coping with the complexity of emotions at the end of life.

67

Family and loved ones: It is important to recognise that the loved ones of patients at the end of life are also profoundly affected emotionally. Offering emotional support to family and friends can help to improve the patient's quality of life by reducing their stress and anxiety.

Recognising the emotional impact of terminal illness is an essential step in providing comprehensive, patient-centred care in palliative care. Healthcare professionals need to create an empathetic and caring environment where patients can safely express their emotions and receive the support they need to cope with the complexity of their feelings.

The Role of the Nurse as Emotional Support

As a nurse, you play a crucial role in providing essential emotional support to patients and their families throughout their end-of-life journey. Your caring, empathetic and compassionate presence helps to create a care environment where emotions can be expressed in confidence and psychological well-being is taken into account.

Active listening and empathy: Active listening and putting yourself in the shoes of the patient and family are key skills in providing emotional support. By listening carefully to their concerns, fears and feelings, you show that you care about their well-being.

Validating emotions: When patients or families express their emotions, it is important to validate them. This means recognising that what they are feeling is normal and understandable in the context of their situation. Validation can help reduce anxiety and promote emotional connection.

Open Communication: Encouraging open and honest communication creates a space where patients and families can share their thoughts and concerns in confidence. This can help identify sources of emotional distress and provide targeted support.

Providing Information: Clearly explaining treatments, care options and processes related to the end of life can help reduce anxiety caused by the unknown. Being informed enables patients and their families to better manage their situation.

Decision Support: Patients and families can be faced with difficult decisions at the end of life. By supporting them in the decision-making process, providing information and respecting their choices, you help to give them a sense of control.

Managing Anxiety and Stress: Stress management skills and relaxation techniques can be useful in helping patients and families manage the anxiety and stress associated with the end of life.

Referral: If necessary, referring patients and families to specialist mental health professionals or support groups can provide more targeted emotional support.

Confidentiality and Respect: By respecting confidentiality and providing a respectful care environment, you create a space where patients and families feel safe to share their emotions.

As a nurse, you are a pillar of emotional support for patients and families at the end of life. Your ability to listen, validate emotions and provide compassionate support plays a crucial role in improving the psychological wellbeing of those you serve, while creating a caring and compassionate care environment.

Promoting the psychological well-being of patients and their families

Promoting the psychological well-being of patients and their families in palliative care is an essential component of overall care. The emotional and psychological challenges associated with the end of life require a caring and sensitive approach to help patients and their families manage stress, develop coping strategies and find comfort.

Needs Assessment: Before psychological well-being can be promoted, it is important to assess the emotional and psychological needs of the patient and their family. This can be done through targeted interviews or questionnaires.

Emotional Support :

- **Empathetic listening:** Offering an attentive and understanding ear to the concerns and emotions of the patient and their family fosters an essential psychological connection and support.
- **Validation of Emotions:** Validating the emotions of the patient and their family by letting them know that what they are feeling is normal and understandable can help reduce anxiety and stress.
- **Professional Support:** Referring patients and their families to specialist mental health professionals, such as psychologists or palliative care counsellors, can offer more targeted emotional support.

Education :
- **Transparent information:** Providing clear and honest information about the disease, treatments and care options can reduce anxiety about the unknown.
- **Awareness of Normal Reactions:** Educating patients and their families about normal emotional reactions at the end of life, such as anticipatory bereavement, can help to normalise their emotions.

Coping strategies :
- **Relaxation techniques:** Teaching relaxation, deep breathing and meditation techniques can help patients and families manage stress and anxiety.
- **Creative expression:** Encouraging the use of creative forms of expression, such as art, music or writing, can help to channel emotions and find an outlet.

Group support :
- **Support groups:** Organising support groups for patients and families can help them share similar experiences, learn from each other and feel less alone in their journey.
- **Online support:** Offering online resources or discussion forums can provide a virtual space for mutual support and information exchange.

Promoting the psychological well-being of patients and their families in palliative care requires a holistic and individualised approach. By providing emotional support, educating about normal reactions and offering practical coping strategies, healthcare professionals help to create a care environment that takes into account the psychological and emotional needs of all those involved.

Depression, Anxiety and Stress Management

Identifying the Signs and Symptoms of Depression

Depression is a major concern in palliative care, as patients at the end of life can be vulnerable to difficult emotional states. Identifying the signs and symptoms of depression is essential to providing adequate psychological support and intervening when necessary. Depression can have a significant impact on a patient's quality of life, and identifying it early enables appropriate care to be provided.

Signs and symptoms :
- **Persistent Sad Mood:** A persistent mood of sadness, hopelessness or emptiness is one of the key symptoms of depression.
- **Loss of interest or pleasure:** Depressed patients may lose interest in activities that used to make them happy.
- **Changes in weight and appetite:** Depression can lead to significant weight loss or gain, as well as a decrease or increase in appetite.
- **Sleep disorders:** Depressed patients may experience sleep problems, such as insomnia or hypersomnia (excessive sleeping).
- **Fatigue and weakness:** Persistent fatigue and reduced energy are common in people with depression.
- **Difficulty concentrating:** Depressed patients may find it difficult to concentrate, make decisions or think clearly.
- **Feelings of uselessness or guilt:** Patients may express feelings of uselessness, excessive guilt or low self-esteem.
- **Thoughts   of death or suicide:** Thoughts of death, suicide or a desire to end one's life are serious warning signs and require immediate intervention.

Assessment and intervention :
- **Full assessment:** When interacting with patients, be alert to signs of depression. Ask open-ended questions about their mood, energy levels and quality of life.
- **Sensitive communication:** If you suspect symptoms of depression, broach the subject sensitively and without judgement. Make sure the patient feels safe to open up to you.
- **Referral to a mental health professional:** If you identify signs of depression, referring the patient to a qualified mental health professional is an important step. An accurate diagnosis and appropriate interventions are needed to help the patient manage depression.
- **Psychological support: As** a nurse, you can also offer emotional support and a sympathetic ear to depressed patients. Your compassionate presence can have a positive impact on their well-being.
- **Working with the care team:** working with doctors, social workers and psychologists to develop a comprehensive treatment plan for the depressed patient.

Early identification of the signs and symptoms of depression is essential for providing appropriate support to patients at the end of life. By remaining vigilant and offering opportunities for emotional expression, you are helping to improve the patient's quality of life by taking into account their psychological well-being.

Therapeutic Approaches to Alleviating Anxiety
Anxiety is common among palliative care patients because of the uncertainties and challenges associated with their condition. Therapeutic approaches aim to help patients manage their anxiety, improve their emotional well-being and offer them strategies for coping with sources of stress. As a nurse, you can play an important role in integrating these approaches into the care you provide.

Relaxation Techniques :
- **Deep breathing:** Teach patients deep breathing techniques to reduce the physical symptoms of anxiety and promote relaxation.
- **Meditation and mindfulness:** Encourage patients to practise meditation and mindfulness to improve their presence in the present moment and reduce anxious ruminations.

Cognitive Behavioural Therapy (CBT) :
- **Identifying Negative Thoughts:** Help patients identify the negative and anxious thoughts that contribute to their anxiety. Once identified, these thoughts can be addressed and reassessed.
- **Development of Management Strategies:** Guide patients in developing strategies to challenge and modify their anxious thoughts, and to adopt a more positive outlook.

Emotional Support :
- **Empathetic listening:** actively listen to patients' concerns and provide a space for them to express their feelings without judgement.
- **Emotion Validation:** Validate patients' emotions by letting them know that what they are feeling is normal and understandable in the context of their situation.

Art therapy :
- **Art therapy:** Encourage patients to take part in artistic activities, such as painting, drawing or writing, to channel their emotions and express their concerns.

Social support :
- **Support groups:** Refer patients to support groups where they can share their experiences and learn from others in similar situations.

Pharmaceutical interventions :
- **Anti-anxiety medication:** If necessary, doctors can prescribe anti-anxiety medication to help reduce anxiety symptoms.

It's important to note that every patient is unique, and what works for one may not work for another. By collaborating with the care team and having open discussions with patients, you can help choose the therapeutic approaches best suited to their needs. By offering emotional support and incorporating anxiety management strategies, you can help to improve the overall well-being of patients at the end of life.

Stress Management Techniques for Patients and Relatives

Stress management is an essential component of palliative care, not only for patients at the end of life but also for their loved ones. The end-of-life period can be emotionally charged and challenging, and helping patients and their families to develop stress management techniques can improve their quality of life and strengthen their ability to cope at this difficult time.

Stress Management Techniques for Patients :
- **Deep breathing:** Teach patients deep breathing techniques to calm the mind and reduce physiological reactions to stress.
- **Meditation and Mindfulness:** Guide patients through meditation and mindfulness exercises to help them focus on the present moment and reduce anxious thoughts.
- **Gentle yoga:** Introducing gentle yoga movements can help release physical and emotional tension, while promoting relaxation.
- **Journaling:** Encourage patients to keep a journal where they can express their emotions, thoughts and concerns.

This can help to clarify their feelings and reduce emotional stress.

Stress Management Techniques for Relatives :

- **Self-care:** Encourage loved ones to take time for themselves by engaging in calming activities such as reading, walking or meditation.
- **Social support:** Direct relatives to support groups or social networks where they can share their experiences and receive support from others in similar situations.
- **Setting limits:** Relatives can feel overwhelmed by their responsibilities. Help them set limits and ask for help when necessary.
- **Communication:** Encourage relatives to communicate openly with patients and with each other to share their concerns and feelings.

Teaching Techniques :

- **Educational sessions:** Organise educational sessions where you teach patients and their families stress management techniques, explaining how and when to use them.
- **Visual support:** Provide visual support, such as brochures or videos, explaining the different stress management techniques.

Customised adaptation :

- **Take preferences into account:** Make sure that the stress management techniques proposed are in line with the individual preferences and beliefs of patients and their families.
- **Reassessment:** Encourage patients and relatives to regularly reassess stress management techniques to determine what works best for them at different stages of their journey.

Stress management is a powerful tool to help patients and their loved ones navigate through the challenges of the end of life. By providing resources, teaching and encouragement to develop these techniques, you are helping to strengthen their ability to cope with stressful times and improve their emotional well-being.

Help with psychological preparation for the end of life

Conversations on Death and End-of-Life Concerns

Conversations about death and end-of-life concerns are often delicate but essential in palliative care. As a nurse, you play an important role in facilitating these discussions with patients and their families. These conversations provide an opportunity to address patients' fears, hopes, values and wishes, which can help create a more appropriate care plan and offer emotional support.

Create a Secure Space :
- **Empathy:** Show empathy and reassure the patient and their family that you are there to support them through these difficult discussions.
- **Non-judgmental: Adopt** a non-judgmental and open attitude, encouraging patients and families to express their thoughts and concerns without fear.

Ask Open Questions:
- **"How are you feeling at the moment?** Ask open-ended questions to give the patient the opportunity to share their feelings and concerns.
- **"Do you have any specific concerns about the end of life?** : Encourage patients to discuss their specific concerns, whether these relate to pain, dignity, spirituality or other important aspects.

Explain the Options :
- **Clarification:** Explain the care options available at the end of life, including palliative care, medical assistance in dying (according to current legislation) and other possible choices.
- **Advanced Care   Planning:** Inform patients of the opportunity to plan their end-of-life care wishes in advance and encourage them to discuss these preferences with their family and care team.

Listen and Respect :
- **Active listening:** Listen carefully to the concerns and wishes expressed by patients and their families.
- **Respecting beliefs:** Respect the patient's cultural, religious and personal beliefs about death and dying.

Supporting families :

- **Include those close to the patient:** Involve those close to the patient in these conversations, as they may also have concerns and questions.
- **Reassure and inform:** Reassure families that these discussions are important to ensure that the patient's wishes are respected and that care is aligned with their values.

Documenting preferences :

- **Care Record:** Clearly document the patient's preferences and wishes regarding end-of-life care in their medical record.
- **Advance Directive:** Encourage patients to write an Advance Care Directive or Advance Declaration in line with local legislation, to ensure that their wishes are respected.

Conversations about death and dying and end-of-life concerns require sensitivity, understanding and active listening. By facilitating these discussions, you enable patients and their families to share their feelings, clarify their wishes and develop a care plan that reflects their values and preferences. This can help create a more respectful and compassionate end-of-life experience for everyone involved.

Support for Patients and Families in the Early Bereavement Phase

Anticipatory bereavement is an emotional process that palliative care patients and their families can go through even before death occurs. As a nurse, you can play a crucial role in providing support to help patients and their families cope with these complex emotions and prepare for the transition to the end of life.

Validation of Emotions :

- **Active listening:** Take the time to listen carefully to the concerns and emotions expressed by patients and their families.
- **Validation:** Validate their emotions by letting them know that anticipatory grief is a normal reaction to the situation and that their feelings are understandable.

Education and Information :
- **Bereavement process:** Explain the concept of anticipatory bereavement and guide patients and their families through the different emotional stages they may experience.
- **Awareness:** Provide information on typical emotions and psychological reactions during this period, to reduce anxiety linked to the unknown.

Emotional expression :
- **Encourage Communication:** Encourage patients and families to openly express their feelings and concerns about the end of life.
- **Creative activities:** Offer creative activities, such as writing, drawing or music, as a means of emotional expression.

Practical preparation :
- **Advanced Care   Planning:** Help patients explore and express their wishes regarding end-of-life care, including preferences for place of death and funeral rites.
- **Managing personal affairs:** Encourage patients to organise their personal affairs, such as making a will, to alleviate concerns about the aftermath of death.

Spiritual support :
- **Religious orientation:** If the patient or family is spiritually oriented, facilitate meetings with spiritual advisers to offer support and advice.

Ongoing support :
- **Regular revisions:** Regularly revisit conversations about anticipatory bereavement to allow patients and their families to express new concerns and emotions.
- **Referral to specialists:** If emotions become overwhelming, refer patients and families to bereavement counsellors or specialist psychologists.

Supporting patients and families in the early stages of bereavement requires a sensitive and compassionate approach. By providing a space for emotional expression, educational information and practical preparation, you help to ease the emotional burden and enable patients and their families to cope better with this period of transition.

Managing Existential and Spiritual Issues at the End of Life
Existential and spiritual issues are often central to the concerns of patients at the end of life. As a nurse, you play a vital role in providing support and openness to discuss these profound issues, which can affect patients' emotional and spiritual well-being.

Creating a Listening Space :
- **Openness:** Provide a warm, non-judgmental space where patients feel comfortable discussing their spiritual and existential questions.
- **Empathetic listening:** Lend an attentive ear to patients' spiritual concerns and offer them the opportunity to share their beliefs and concerns.

Discussions on Beliefs :
- **Spiritual issues:** Encourage patients to discuss their spiritual beliefs, whether religious, philosophical or existential.
- **Impact on End of Life:** Help patients explore how their beliefs influence their perceptions of death and end of life.

Spiritual orientation :
- **Religious support:** If patients are religiously affiliated, facilitate their access to spiritual advisors or members of the clergy to offer advice and support.
- **Exploring Spirituality:** Encourage patients to explore their spirituality, even if they are not affiliated with a specific religion. This may include meditation, contemplation or connecting with nature.

Existential Questions :
- **Meaning of life:** Facilitate discussions about the meaning of life, the achievements, relationships and lessons that have shaped their journey.
- **Achievement and Regrets:** Help patients reflect on what they have achieved in their lives and deal with any regrets.

Facilitating Reconciliation:
- **Conflict resolution:** If there are conflicts with people close to them, encourage patients to consider reconciliation and express their feelings.

Spirituality and Dignity :
- **Reinforcing Dignity:** Help patients see how spirituality can reinforce their sense of dignity at the end of life and help them cope with the challenges.

- **Acceptance and letting go:** Encourage patients to explore how their spiritual or existential beliefs can contribute to acceptance and letting go.

As a nurse, your role in managing existential and spiritual issues is to provide a space for discussion and support, regardless of patients' beliefs. By showing empathy and encouraging exploration, you help patients find answers and meaning in their own spiritual and existential journey at the end of life.

Chapter 6:
Communication and Ethics
in Palliative Care

Communication with Patients and Families

Establishing an Open Communications Environment

Open communication is at the heart of palliative care, fostering trust, understanding and well-being for both patients and their families. As a nurse, you play a key role in creating an environment conducive to honest and open communication, where patients and their families can freely express their concerns, needs and wishes.

Creating a welcoming climate :
- **Empathy:** Show empathy towards patients and families, demonstrating that you are there to listen and understand them.
- **Non-judgemental:** Adopt a non-judgmental attitude, encouraging patients and families to express themselves without fear of being criticised.

Using Accessible Languages :
- **Avoid complex medical terms:** Use simple, understandable language to explain medical information and care options.
- **Repeat and summarise:** Repeat or summarise important information to make sure patients and families understand.

Encouraging participation :
- **Ask Open Questions:** Ask questions that encourage patients and families to share their concerns and views.
- **Listen Actively:** Pay attention to what patients and families are saying, and show that you take them seriously.

Patient Empowerment :
- **Informed Decision Making:** Provide patients with the information they need to actively participate in making decisions about their care.
- **Respect Choices:** Respect patients' choices, even if they differ from what you suggest, recognising that it is their life and their decision.

Ensuring confidentiality:
- **Respect for privacy:** Choose appropriate times for confidential discussions and make sure that patients feel comfortable talking in private.

Inform about the Roles :
- **Roles of the team:** Inform patients and families of the roles and responsibilities of the members of the palliative care team so that they know who to contact.
- **Listening role:** Present yourself as someone with whom they can discuss their concerns and ask questions.

Supporting Friends and Family :
- **Inclusion of Relatives:** Encourage relatives to take part in discussions and express their concerns, as they are also part of the care team.
- **Coordination:** Ensure that information is shared with relatives with the patient's consent, so that they are informed and supported.

By creating an environment of open communication, you lay a solid foundation for patient- and family-centred palliative care. Your ability to listen carefully, respect choices and provide clear information helps to build trust and facilitate informed decision-making.

Strategies for Explaining the Medical Situation Sensitively
Explaining the medical situation sensitively is a crucial skill in palliative care. When communicating medical information to patients and their families, it is important to do so in a way that is understandable and caring, while taking into account their emotions and needs.

Creating a Comfortable Environment:
- **Choice of location:** Choose a quiet, private place to discuss the medical situation, where patients and families can feel at ease.
- **Empathetic attitude:** Demonstrate an empathetic attitude from the outset, showing that you are there to support them.

Using understandable language :
- **Avoid Technical Terms:** Avoid complex medical terms and use simple language to explain the medical situation.

- **Analogies and Comparisons:** Use analogies or comparisons to make medical explanations more understandable.

Answering Questions :

- **Encourage questions:** Encourage patients and families to ask questions at any time and make sure they answer honestly.
- **Take your time:** Take the time you need to answer questions thoroughly and accurately.

Communicating Care Options :

- **Presentation of Options:** Explain the different care options available depending on the medical situation, highlighting the advantages and disadvantages.
- **Care Plan:** Work with the patient and their family to develop a care plan that respects their choices and values.

Respecting emotions :

- **Emotional reactions:** Be prepared to deal with emotional reactions, such as anger, sadness or shock, by providing support and reassurance.
- **Emotion Validation:** Validate the emotions expressed by patients and their families, showing that their feelings are understandable.

Using visual aids :

- **Graphs and diagrams:** Use simple graphs or diagrams to illustrate medical concepts in a visual way.
- **Informative brochures:** Provide informative brochures or documents to enable patients and their families to review information at their own pace.

Coordinate with the Team :

- **Consistency of information:** Make sure that the information you provide is consistent with that provided by other members of the care team.
- **Specialist resources:** If the medical situation is complex, refer patients and their families to specialists or medical advisers for more detailed explanations.

Explaining the medical situation sensitively requires an approach that is patient, compassionate and tailored to individual needs. By taking emotions into account, providing clear explanations and offering care options, you help patients and their families to better understand their situation and make informed decisions for their palliative care journey.

Helping Patients to Understand and Accept their Health Condition

Helping patients to understand and accept their condition in palliative care requires sensitive and empathetic communication. You play a key role in providing honest information and supporting patients through the process of awareness and acceptance.

Explain clearly:
- **Use of Analogies:** Use analogies or comparisons to simplify medical explanations and make the situation more understandable.
- **Avoid medical jargon:** Avoid using complex medical language and ensure that explanations are adapted to the patient's level of understanding.

Listen to the reactions :
- **Active listening:** Listen carefully to the patient's reactions and questions, providing a space for them to express their feelings and concerns.
- **Responding to emotions:** Respond to the patient's emotions with understanding, showing that you recognise their concerns.

Providing Resources :
- **Informative material:** Provide informative brochures, documents or videos so that patients can learn more at their own pace.
- **Link to specialists:** If necessary, refer patients to specialists or advisers who can provide more detailed information about their condition.

Explain the Care Options :
- **Discussion of Choices:** Explain the different care options available depending on the medical situation, highlighting the advantages and disadvantages.
- **Include Loved Ones:** Encourage patients to discuss their care options with their loved ones in order to make an informed decision.

Supporting the Stages of Grief :
- **Denial and anger:** Understand that patients may go through stages of denial and anger about their condition. Offer emotional support during these times.
- **Negotiation and Acceptance:** Help patients explore ways of adapting their understanding of the situation and moving towards acceptance.

83

Promoting independence :
- **Decision-making:** Encourage patients to make decisions based on their preferences and values, while informing them of the implications.
- **Pressure-free advice:** Offer advice and information without putting pressure on patients to make specific decisions.

Ongoing monitoring :
- **Regular review:** Go back over the discussions to check the patient's understanding, answer new questions and adapt the explanations as their understanding evolves.

Helping patients to understand and accept their condition requires patience and empathy. By providing clear information, listening attentively and offering emotional support, you accompany them on their journey of understanding and acceptance, which can contribute to a more serene and respectful end-of-life experience.

Shared decision-making and advance directives

Importance of Informed Decision Making

Informed decision-making is at the heart of palliative care, enabling patients to play an active role in their own care pathway. As a nurse, you have a vital role to play in helping patients understand their options, providing detailed information and supporting them to make decisions that reflect their values and preferences.

Respect for autonomy :
- **Right to Information:** Inform patients of their right to know the details of their condition, treatment options and their implications.
- **Active role:** Encourage patients to take an active role in making decisions about their care, based on their preferences and values.

Understanding Options :
- **Detailed explanations:** Provide clear, detailed explanations of the different treatment options, using accessible language.

- **Advantages and disadvantages:** Discuss the advantages and disadvantages of each option, taking into account medical considerations and patient preferences.

Involvement of family and friends :

- **Inclusion of Families:** Include the patient's family in decision-making discussions, as they can offer additional support and perspective.
- **Consensus:** Encourage patients and their families to work together to reach a consensus on care choices.

Consideration of Values and Preferences :

- **Values Discussion:** Explore the patient's personal values and how they influence their end-of-life care preferences.
- **Life context:** Understand the patient's life context, including religious, cultural and family beliefs, to guide decisions.

Advanced Care Planning :

- **Advance directives :** Discuss the possibility of the patient writing advance directives to express their wishes regarding future care.
- **Trusted Person:** Encourage patients to appoint a trusted person to make medical decisions on their behalf if necessary.

Ongoing assessment :

- **Regular Review:** Revisit decisions made periodically, taking into account changes in the patient's state of health and changing preferences.
- **Adaptation:** Be prepared to adapt care plans as the situation and the patient's wishes evolve.

Informed decision-making allows patients to remain in control of their care journey, taking into account their values and preferences. By helping patients understand their options and facilitating open discussions, you help create a patient-centred end-of-life experience that respects their wishes.

Involving patients and their families in care decisions

Involving the patient and family in care decisions is an essential practice in palliative care. As a nurse, you play a key role in facilitating open discussions and promoting collaboration between the patient, their family and the care team, to ensure that care choices are aligned with the patient's values, preferences and needs.

Creating an Inclusive Environment:
- **Family meetings:** Organise family meetings to discuss care options and allow all members to share their views.
- **Encouraging expression: Make sure that** every member of the family feels encouraged to express their concerns and opinions.

Sharing information :
- **Clear explanations:** Provide clear information about the patient's medical situation, using language that is accessible to all family members.
- **Care Options:** Explain in detail the different care options available, highlighting the advantages and disadvantages of each choice.

Facilitating decision-making :
- **Guided Discussions:** Facilitate open discussions by asking open-ended questions that allow the patient and family to express their preferences and concerns.
- **Balancing voices:** Make sure that the patient's voice is taken into account and balanced with those of family members.

Consider Values and Preferences :
- **Individual interviews:** If necessary, organise individual interviews with the patient and each family member to understand their values and preferences.
- **Respectful approach: Take** everyone's religious, cultural and personal beliefs into account when making decisions.

Working with the care team:
- **Coordination:** Work with other members of the care team to ensure that all information is shared and care options are understood.
- **Referrals:** If complex decisions need to be made, refer the patient and family to medical advisers or specialists for further advice.

Setting Care Objectives :
- **Patient priorities:** Identify the patient's and family's care objectives, whether these relate to pain management, quality of life or other aspects.
- **Personalised Care Plan:** Draw up a personalised care plan that takes account of each person's goals and preferences.

Involving the patient and their family in care decisions ensures that the care plan is patient-centred and reflects their needs and values. By facilitating open discussions and encouraging collaboration, you create an environment where the patient and their family feel supported and listened to, contributing to a more respectful and meaningful end-of-life experience.

Use of Advance Directives and Living Wills
Advance directives and living wills are important tools in palliative care to help patients express their wishes about their future care and end of life. As a nurse, you can play a vital role in informing patients and their families about these documents and helping them to draw them up, ensuring that their choices are respected even if they are unable to express their wishes afterwards.

Advance directives :
- **Definition:** Explain to patients and families what advance directives are, which are legal documents that allow patients to indicate in advance the care they wish to receive or refuse in the event of incapacity to communicate.
- **Content:** Help patients understand the different care options, such as resuscitation, artificial feeding, etc., and choose those that correspond to their values.
- **Registration:** Explain how to register advance directives with the relevant authorities and how to share them with the care team.

Living Wills :
- **Definition:** Inform patients and their families about living wills, which are narrative documents that allow patients to share their values, beliefs and care preferences.
- **Content:** Help patients to think about and write down their life stories, their care preferences and what is important to them.
- **Use:** Explain how living wills can guide care decisions and how they can be shared with the care team and relatives.

Facilitating Conversation :
- **Open Discussion:** Encourage patients to discuss their care preferences with their loved ones and to include these discussions in their advance directives or living will.
- **Exploring Values:** Help patients reflect on the values that guide their care choices, particularly at the end of life.

Coordination with the Care Team :
- • **Document Sharing:** Ensure that advance directives and living wills are included in the patient's medical record and shared with other members of the care team.
- • **Regular Review:** Encourage patients to review and update their advance directives and living wills as their preferences and health status change.

The use of advance directives and living wills gives patients the power to control their future care and ensure that their choices are respected. By explaining these documents, helping to develop them and coordinating their use with the care team, you ensure that patients' wishes are respected throughout their palliative care journey.

Ethical Dilemmas and Patient Values

Addressing Ethical Dilemmas in Palliative Care
Palliative care is often accompanied by complex ethical dilemmas, given the difficult choices that can arise at the end of life. As a nurse, it is essential to recognise and address these dilemmas in an ethical and respectful manner, bearing in mind the patient's well-being, preferences and rights.

Dilemma recognition :
- • **Sensitivity to Complex Situations:** Be attentive to situations where care choices may be conflicting or difficult, paying attention to the patient's values and preferences.
- • **Consultation with the Care Team:** Hold regular discussions with members of the care team to share perspectives and advice on managing ethical dilemmas.

Ethical decision-making :
- • **Patient autonomy:** Respect the patient's right to make informed decisions and ensure that they are informed of all available options.
- • **Beneficence:** Ensure that care choices promote the patient's well-being and quality of life.
- • **Non-maleficence:** Avoid causing unnecessary harm to the patient and take account of their treatment preferences.

Open Communication:
- **Multidisciplinary discussion:** Discuss ethical dilemmas with the care team, including doctors, social workers and counsellors, to obtain a variety of perspectives.
- **Patient Inclusion:** Engage in open communication with the patient and family to discuss ethical dilemmas and their implications.

Respect for Values and Beliefs :
- **Consideration of Values: Take into account** the patient's religious, cultural and personal values when making ethical decisions.
- **External consultation:** If the ethical dilemma is complex, consider consulting medical ethicists or ethics committees for advice and recommendations.

Documenting decisions :
- **Complete records:** Document the discussions and decisions taken concerning ethical dilemmas, ensuring that everything is clearly recorded in the patient's medical file.
- **Rationale:** Include the reasoning behind the decisions taken, showing that ethical considerations have been taken into account.

Emotional Support :
- **Support for the team:** Offer emotional support to the care team, as managing ethical dilemmas can be emotionally challenging.
- **Patient support:** Offer emotional support to patients and their families during the decision-making process, helping them to understand the options and implications.

Managing ethical dilemmas in palliative care requires a thoughtful and collaborative approach. By approaching these situations with sensitivity, taking ethical principles into account and involving the patient and the care team, you help to create an environment where decisions are made in the patient's best interests and with respect for their values and wishes.

Respecting the patient's religious and cultural beliefs

Respect for the patient's religious and cultural beliefs is of paramount importance in palliative care, as it ensures that care is tailored to individual values and preferences. As a nurse, you play a key role in ensuring that care respects patients' religious beliefs and practices, as well as their cultural customs.

Continuing Education :
- **Familiarisation with Cultures:** Learn the basics of the most common religious and cultural beliefs and practices in order to better understand patients' needs.
- **Consultation with experts:** If necessary, consult religious and cultural resources or advisers to better understand specific needs.

Open Communication:
- **Early discussion:** From the outset, engage in open discussions about the patient's religious and cultural beliefs to understand how these may influence their care preferences.
- **Open questions:** Ask open-ended questions to allow patients to express their concerns and preferences related to their beliefs.

Personalised care :
- **Individual Care Plan:** Develop a care plan that is adapted to the patient's religious and cultural beliefs, ensuring that it is respectful and meaningful.
- **Funeral customs:** Find out about specific funeral customs and make sure you respect them in the event of the patient's death.

Food and Religious Rituals :
- **Diets:** Respect specific diets dictated by the patient's religious beliefs, ensuring that meals are in line with their practices.
- **Religious rituals:** Provide space and support for the patient to practise religious rituals, such as prayer or meditation.

Observance of the Holy Days :
- **Adapting care:** If the patient observes specific holy days, adapt care accordingly to take account of these requirements.
- **Pre-consultation:** Talk to the patient and their family to understand the adjustments needed during religious holidays.

Confidentiality and Respect :
- **Protecting confidentiality:** Ensure that patients' religious and cultural information is treated with the utmost respect and confidentiality.

- **Respectful approach:** Show respect for the patient's religious objects and symbols, avoiding any insensitive attitude or comment.

Respect for the patient's religious and cultural beliefs is fundamental to providing quality palliative care. By establishing open communication, adapting care to specific needs and showing respect for religious and cultural practices, you create an environment where the patient feels understood and supported, which contributes to a respectful and patient-centred end-of-life experience.

Ethical Conflicts: Collaboration with the Medical Team and the Family

Managing ethical conflicts in palliative care can be particularly tricky because of the complexity of the situations and the emotions involved. As a nurse, your role is to facilitate collaboration between the medical team, the patient's family and other stakeholders, in order to find solutions that respect everyone's values and needs.

Early recognition :
- **Awareness:** Be vigilant for early signs of ethical conflict, such as disagreements over treatment options or a patient's end-of-life preferences.
- **Openness to Communication:** Create an environment where members of the medical team and the patient's family feel comfortable expressing their concerns.

Transparent communication :
- **Information sharing:** Ensure that all stakeholders are fully and accurately informed about the medical situation and treatment options.
- **Active listening:** Listen carefully to the concerns of the medical team and the family, showing empathy and understanding.

Multidisciplinary meeting :
- **Inclusion of the medical team:** Organise meetings with doctors, nurses, social workers and other healthcare professionals to discuss treatment options and ethical dilemmas openly.

- **Exchanging perspectives:** Encourage each team member to share their perspective, taking into account different points of view.

Facilitating Mediation :

- **Role of Mediator:** If the conflict persists, consider involving a neutral mediator to facilitate communication and resolution.
- **Foster mutual respect:** Help stakeholders focus on the patient's interests and find solutions that respect the patient's wishes and values.

Ethics and Clinical Practice :

- **Alignment with Ethical Principles:** Ensure that decisions taken are aligned with the ethical principles of beneficence, non-maleficence, autonomy and justice.
- **Consultation with Experts:** If necessary, seek the advice of medical ethicists or ethics committees for further guidance.

Emotional Support :

- **Family support:** Offer emotional support to the patient's family, helping them to understand treatment options and ethical considerations.
- **Stress management:** You should also offer emotional support to the medical team, as managing ethical conflicts can be stressful.

Managing ethical conflicts requires a collaborative approach and open communication. By promoting transparency, facilitating multidisciplinary discussions and seeking solutions that respect the values and needs of all stakeholders, you help to create an environment where ethical dilemmas are addressed in a constructive, patient-centred manner.

Chapter 7:
Support for Families and Friends

The Crucial Role of Families in Palliative Care

Recognising the Central Role of Relatives in the Care Process

Relatives play an essential role in the palliative care process, as they are often the main carers and emotional supporters of patients at the end of life. As a nurse, it is crucial to recognise and respect the central role that relatives play and to work closely with them to ensure the patient's overall well-being.

Assessment of the role of close relations :

- **Raising awareness:** Be aware of the importance of relatives as key members of the care and support team for patients at the end of life.
- **Acknowledgement:** Express your gratitude to the people close to you for their commitment and dedication to the patient's well-being.

Listening and Communication :

- **Active listening:** Take the time to listen carefully to the concerns, questions and needs of those close to the patient.
- **Open communication:** Provide transparent information about the patient's condition, care options and decisions, encouraging relatives to ask questions.

Collaboration and Information Sharing :

- **Shared decision-making:** Involve family members in decision-making about the patient's care, taking into account their preferences and those of the patient.
- **Coordination:** Work closely with relatives to coordinate the patient's care and needs, maintaining regular communication.

Emotional Support :

- **Support for loved ones:** Offer emotional support to those close to the patient, as they may feel stress, anxiety and sadness during this difficult period.

- **Empathetic listening:** Be empathetic towards the emotions of loved ones and provide a safe space for them to express their feelings.

Training and Education :

- **Care information:** Educate loved ones about palliative care, pain management, symptoms and available care options.
- **Practical elements:** Explain practical tasks, such as administering medication, so that relatives feel competent and confident.

Inclusion in Care :

- **Assistance with Daily Care:** Encourage relatives to participate in the patient's daily care, such as personal hygiene and feeding.
- **Comfort and presence:** Allow family members to stay with the patient to provide comfort and companionship.

Recognising the central role of relatives in the palliative care process reinforces the holistic approach to care and ensures a more sustained experience for the patient. By working in partnership with loved ones, you create an environment where the patient's family and friends feel included and respected, contributing to a more dignified and meaningful end-of-life experience.

The Emotional Impact of Palliative Care on Families

Palliative care has a profound emotional impact on the families of patients at the end of life, as they face emotional, psychological and practical challenges throughout the process. As a nurse, it is important to recognise and respond to this emotional impact, offering caring support and helping families to cope with the challenges that arise.

Shock and Denial :

- **Understanding the process:** Recognise that families may experience initial shock and difficulty in accepting the reality of terminal illness.
- **Emotional support:** Offer a space for families to express their emotions and provide empathic support during this difficult phase.

Guilt and Anger:
- **Feelings of guilt:** Understand that families may feel guilty for not having been able to prevent the illness or for not being able to provide all the necessary care.
- **Anger Management:** Offer advice on dealing with anger and frustration, encouraging healthy ways of releasing these emotions.

Anxiety and Worry :
- **Uncertainty:** Recognise that families may feel anxious about the uncertainty of the future and the rapid changes in the patient's state of health.
- **Information and education:** Provide clear information about the illness, care options and expectations, to reduce anxiety.

Anticipated bereavement:
- **Bereavement process:** Understand that families may begin an early bereavement process while the patient is still alive, which can be emotionally complex.
- **Bereavement support:** Offer support in dealing with these emotions and explain that anticipatory grief is a normal reaction.

Impact on Family Dynamics :
- **Adjustments:** Recognise that family roles and dynamics may change as the family supports the patient at the end of life.
- **Communication:** Encourage open communication between family members to resolve conflicts and preserve bonds.

Self-care for Families :
- **Encouraging self-care:** Remind families of the importance of taking care of themselves during this stressful time, by offering advice on how to manage their own well-being.
- **Support Resources:** Refer families to support groups, counsellors or resources to help them cope with their own emotional impact.

Recognising the emotional impact of palliative care on families is key to providing holistic support. By offering emotional support, clear information and stress management resources, you help families navigate the emotional challenges of their loved one's end of life, contributing to a more comforting and meaningful experience for all family members.

Working with Families to Deliver Optimal Care

Working with families is essential to providing optimal care in palliative care, as they bring valuable knowledge about the patient, their preferences and their history. As a nurse, working in partnership with families helps to create a more comprehensive, patient-centred care plan.

Establishing a relationship of trust :
- **Warm welcome:** Create a welcoming and reassuring environment for families, so that they feel comfortable sharing their concerns.
- **Active listening:** Practice attentive and respectful listening to show families that their voices are heard.

Information sharing :
- **Transparency:** Share relevant information about the patient's state of health, treatment options and goals of care.
- **Continuing Education:** Provide educational information on palliative care, symptom management and available resources.

Collaborative planning :
- **Inclusion of Patient Preferences:** Involve families in drawing up the care plan, taking into account the patient's preferences and values.
- **Ongoing adjustments:** Work with families to adjust the care plan in line with the patient's changing state of health.

Care Coordination :
- **Transition management:** Work with families to facilitate transitions between different levels of care and medical facilities.
- **Active participation:** Encourage families to be active partners in the coordination of care, ensuring that information is shared between all care providers.

Emotional and Practical Support :
- **Bereavement support:** Offer empathetic support in the event of bereavement in advance and after the patient's death, by providing resources for bereavement support.
- **Practical guidance:** Refer families to resources to help them navigate the practical aspects of palliative care and bereavement.

Taking into account the needs of the family :
- **Listening to needs:** Ask families about their specific needs in terms of emotional support, resources and information.
- **Adapting Care:** Use the information provided by families to adapt care to the overall needs of the patient and their family.

Working with families enriches the palliative care experience by creating a patient-centred care partnership. By working together to develop care plans, provide emotional support and coordinate care, you help create an environment where families feel supported and patients benefit from a more holistic and comfortable end-of-life experience.

Accompaniment and Emotional Support for Loved Ones

Providing Emotional Support in Times of Stress
Families of palliative care patients often go through periods of intense emotional stress. As a nurse, you have an important role to play in providing compassionate emotional support and helping families cope with these difficult times.

Empathic Presence :
- **Be present:** Offer your attentive and compassionate presence to the families, showing that you are there to support them.
- **Active listening:** Listen actively to their concerns, emotions and worries, without judgement.

Validation of Emotions :
- **Validation:** Validate families' emotions by showing them that their reactions are normal in stressful situations such as these.
- **Empathy:** Show empathy by expressing your understanding and sympathy for what they are going through.

Comfort and Practical Support :
- **Emotional support:** Offer words of comfort and support to help families through their time of distress.

- **Practical support:** Offer help with practical and organisational tasks that can add to stress, such as coordinating care or finding resources.

Referral to Resources :
- **Support groups:** Refer families to support groups or therapists who specialise in palliative care.
- **Counsellors and therapists:** Encourage families to seek the help of a counsellor or therapist for professional emotional support.

Managing Anxiety :
- **Stress Management Techniques:** Teaching breathing, relaxation and meditation techniques to help families manage their anxiety.
- **Mindfulness practices:** Show how mindfulness can help reduce stress by focusing on the present moment.

Encouraging Personal Care:
- **Self-care:** Remind families of the importance of taking care of themselves by engaging in activities that nourish them emotionally.
- **Breaks and rest:** Encourage families to take regular breaks to avoid emotional exhaustion.

Providing emotional support in times of stress is a crucial part of palliative care. By offering empathic support, practical advice and stress management resources, you can help families cope better with intense emotions and maintain emotional balance during this difficult time.

Offering Resources to Help Loved Ones Cope

The relatives of palliative care patients often need resources to help them cope with the emotional and practical challenges of this period. As a nurse, you can play an important role in providing information and referrals to appropriate resources.

Information material :
- **Brochures and leaflets:** Provide brochures and leaflets that explain palliative care, common symptoms and available support resources.
- **Practical guides:** Offer practical guides on how to care for a patient at the end of life, including information on basic care and symptom management.

Support groups :
- **Referral to groups:** Inform family members about local support groups where they can meet other people with similar experiences.
- **Online Groups:** Present online forums and discussion groups where loved ones can connect with others in similar situations.

Advisors and Therapists:
- **Professional Referrals:** Provide referrals to specialist palliative care counsellors and therapists for professional emotional support.
- **Advice on Selection:** Give advice on how to choose an appropriate mental health professional.

Self-care resources :
- **Stress Management Techniques:** Teach relaxation, breathing and meditation techniques to help loved ones manage their own stress.
- **Well-being activities:** Offer wellness activities, such as yoga or walking, to help loved ones maintain their own mental health.

Institutions and Associations :
- **Referrals:** Refer relatives to organisations and associations that specialise in palliative care, offering information and support.
- **Helplines:** Provide the telephone numbers of mental health helplines, where loved ones can get support if they need it urgently.

Bereavement resources :
- **Bereavement literature:** Offer books and online resources on the bereavement process to help loved ones anticipate and manage their grief.
- **Bereavement Support Groups:** Inform relatives about local bereavement support groups where they can find support after the patient's death.

Providing resources to help relatives cope is an essential aspect of palliative care. By offering information, guidance and advice on managing emotional stress, you are helping to build the resilience of loved ones and helping them to get through this difficult time with the tools and knowledge at their disposal.

Listening to and Validating the Emotions of Bereaved Families

The bereavement process is a complex emotional time for families who have lost a loved one in palliative care. As a nurse, it is crucial to provide a space for listening to and validating the emotions that families may be feeling during this difficult time.

Active listening :
- **Attentive presence:** Offer your presence and undivided attention to bereaved families, being available to listen whenever they need it.
- **Non-judgmental:** Create a safe environment where families feel comfortable expressing themselves without fear of being judged.

Validation of Emotions :
- **Empathy:** Show empathy by recognising families' emotions and expressing that their feelings are legitimate.
- **Validation:** Use phrases such as "I understand you feel that way" to validate the emotions they share.

Encouraging self-expression :
- **Open to Conversation:** Encourage families to express their emotions, memories and concerns freely.
- **Sharing Experiences:** If appropriate, share personal stories to create a sense of connection and mutual understanding.

Avoid clichés:
- **Avoid platitudes:** Avoid using ready-made phrases such as "it's for the best" or "time will heal everything", as they can minimise families' emotions.
- **Deep listening:** Focus on listening rather than giving quick answers, allowing families to feel truly heard.

Respecting the Progression of Mourning :
- **Listening over time:** Be prepared to listen to bereaved families at different points in their journey, as their emotions may change over time.
- **Adapting your approach:** Tailor your approach to the specific emotions that families share at different stages of bereavement.

Referrals to Professional Support :
- **Bereavement counsellors:** If necessary, recommend specialist bereavement counsellors for professional emotional support.

- **Bereavement support groups:** Refer families to bereavement support groups where they can share their emotions with others facing a similar loss.

Listening to and validating the emotions of bereaved families is an essential aspect of palliative care. By providing a safe space for emotional expression and showing empathy, you help families cope with their grief and find comfort during this difficult time.

Managing Family Conflicts and Interpersonal Dynamics

Identifying and Managing Potential Conflicts within the Family

Families in palliative care can experience emotional tension and conflict due to the pressure of the situation and the intense emotions linked to the end of life of a loved one. As a nurse, it is important to recognise and manage these conflicts to maintain a supportive and collaborative environment.

Signs of Conflict :
- **Difficult communication:** Identify communication difficulties, frequent arguments or a lack of cooperation between family members.
- **Visible tensions:** Watch out for signs of emotional tension or obvious disagreements in your interactions with the family.

Listening and Validation :
- **Active listening:** Provide a space for family members to express their concerns and points of view.
- **Validate emotions:** Validate everyone's emotions and perspectives, showing that you understand their point of view.

Mediation :
- **Role of Mediator:** If necessary and with the agreement of the parties, act as a mediator to facilitate communication between family members.
- **Balance:** Make sure that every member of the family has the opportunity to express their views and be heard.

Expectation Management :
- **Clarifying Expectations:** Help clarify each family member's expectations of care, medical decisions and respective roles.
- **Open communication:** Encourage open and honest communication to avoid misunderstandings.

Reminder of the Common Objective :
- **Patient-centred:** Remind the family that the common goal is the patient's well-being at the end of life, and that conflict can be counter-productive.
- **Priority to Quality of Life:** Stress the importance of preserving the patient's quality of life and dignity at this time.

References to External Support :
- **Family counsellors:** Refer the family to family counsellors or therapists who can help them manage conflicts.
- **Professional intervention:** If conflicts persist, recommend the intervention of a mental health professional to help resolve them.

Confidentiality :
- **Respecting confidentiality:** Assure family members that their discussions and concerns will be treated confidentially.
- **Professional limitations:** Explain your limitations as a nurse and offer help in directing them to the appropriate resources.

Managing conflict within the family in palliative care can be complex, but it is essential to maintaining an environment of support and mutual understanding. By recognising the signs of conflict, encouraging open communication and offering resources for mediation, you help to maintain harmony within the family and ensure that the patient receives the best possible care during this delicate period.

Facilitating Communication and Conflict Resolution

As a nurse, facilitating communication and conflict resolution within the family is a crucial aspect of your role. Effective conflict management helps to create an optimal supportive environment for the patient at the end of life and their loved ones.

Creating an Open Communication Space :
- **Family meetings:** Organise regular family meetings to discuss care, medical decisions and emotional concerns.
- **Active listening:** Practice attentive listening during group discussions, encouraging each member of the family to express themselves.

Using Communication Techniques :
- **Paraphrase:** Repeat each other's concerns to make sure you understand correctly.
- **Empathy:** Show empathy by expressing that you understand everyone's emotions and perspectives.

Encouraging collaboration :
- **Focus on the patient:** Regularly remind yourself that the patient at the end of life is the priority, which can help to put disagreements aside.
- **Finding Shared Solutions:** Encourage the family to work together to find solutions that work for everyone.

Establishing Communication Rules :
- **Mutual respect:** Establish communication rules that encourage mutual respect, even in the event of disagreement.
- **Avoid blame:** Encourage the family to avoid blaming other members and to focus on solutions.

Conflict intervention :
- **Mediation:** If the conflict persists, offer to act as a mediator to facilitate conversation between family members.
- **Maintain neutrality:** During mediation, maintain a neutral position and make sure that each party feels heard.

Developing communication skills :
- **Training:** Offer communication training sessions to family members, focusing on active listening and conflict resolution.
- **Repeat Key Messages:** Repeat key messages to ensure that the information is understood and integrated.

Keeping the Patient Informed:
- **Transparency:** Inform patients about family discussions that concern them, while respecting their confidentiality preferences.
- **Inclusion of the patient:** If the patient wishes, include him/her in family discussions so that he/she can express his/her concerns.

Facilitating communication and conflict resolution within the family requires sensitive communication skills and a patient approach. By encouraging openness, collaboration and mutual respect, you help to create an environment conducive to making informed decisions and maintaining harmonious relationships during this emotionally charged time.

Ongoing Support to Preserve Family Relationships

Preserving family relationships during palliative care is essential to ensure the well-being of the patient at the end of life and the emotional support of their loved ones. As a nurse, you can play a crucial role in providing ongoing support to maintain strong and harmonious family relationships.

Raising awareness of the importance of family relationships :
- **Discussion:** Talk to the family about the importance of solidarity and cooperation in these difficult times.
- **Strengthening ties:** Remind families that strong bonds can bring comfort to the patient and loved ones.

Education on Bereavement and Emotions :
- **Open communication:** Encourage families to express their emotions and discuss their concerns honestly.
- **Normalising Grief:** Explain that different people may react differently to bereavement and that this can affect relationships.

Encouraging ongoing communication :
- **Regular meetings:** Organise regular family meetings to discuss care, decisions and concerns.
- **Active listening:** Promote attentive listening and encourage each member of the family to share their opinions and concerns.

Preventing misunderstandings :
- **Clarifying information:** Ensure that information about medical care and decisions is clearly understood by all family members.
- **Repeating Key Information:** Repeat important information to make sure everyone understands it.

Strengthening Positive Roles:
- **Highlighting strengths:** Identify and encourage the strengths and skills of each family member to boost their confidence.

- **Assigning roles:** Involve family members in care and tasks according to their skills and preferences.

References to External Resources :

- **Family counsellors:** Refer families to family counsellors or therapists specialising in relationship management.
- **Support groups:** Inform families about support groups for relatives of palliative care patients.

Creation of a Support Environment :

- **Listening and support:** Show that you are available to listen to families' concerns and offer advice when needed.
- **Neutrality:** Be neutral and fair in your interactions with all family members to avoid favouring certain members.

Preserving family relationships during palliative care requires ongoing support and open communication. By encouraging listening, mutual understanding and harmony, you help to create an environment where families feel supported, which is essential for the well-being of the patient at the end of life and to help loved ones through this difficult period.

Chapter 8:
Comfort and End-of-Life Care

Preparation for the end of life and comfort care

Exploring the Expectations and Preferences of Patients at the End of Life

Exploring the patient's expectations and preferences at the end of life is an essential aspect of palliative care. As a nurse, your role is to create a safe and respectful space where the patient can express their wishes, needs and concerns for end-of-life care. This is crucial to providing personalised care that respects the patient's dignity and quality of life.

Creating a Favourable Environment :
- **Confidentiality:** Make sure the environment is private and that the patient feels confident to share their thoughts and preferences.
- **Empathy:** Show empathy and sensitivity towards the patient, demonstrating that you are there to listen and support them.

Encouraging the expression of expectations:
- **Open questions:** Ask open-ended questions to encourage patients to share their expectations, wishes and concerns.
- **Take the time:** Give patients enough time to think and express themselves, without feeling rushed.

Explore Care and Comfort:
- **Medical treatments:** Discuss the treatment options available and the goals of care based on the patient's situation.
- **Comfort Care:** Explain palliative and end-of-life care options to help patients understand the choices available to them.

Discuss Location Preferences :
- **Place of Care:** Ask if the patient has any preferences as to where they would like to receive their palliative care, whether at home, in a hospice or in hospital.

- **Family environment:** Find out whether the patient wishes to be surrounded by family and friends during this period.

Exploring Values and Beliefs :
- **Spiritual beliefs:** If the patient has spiritual beliefs, discuss how these may influence their wishes for end-of-life care.
- **Personal Values:** Explore the patient's personal values and how they can guide care decisions.

Registration of decisions :
- **Document Preferences:** Make sure you record the patient's preferences and wishes in their medical record to inform future decisions.
- **Legal documents:** If the patient wishes, discuss the drafting of legal documents such as advance directives and living wills.

Exploring a patient's expectations and preferences at the end of life requires a sensitive and respectful approach. By establishing open communication, asking pertinent questions and listening attentively, you can help the patient express their wishes and make informed decisions about their end-of-life care. This helps to honour the patient's dignity and provide care that respects their values and choices.

Creating a Comfortable and Soothing Environment

Creating a comfortable and soothing environment is an essential aspect of palliative care for patients at the end of life. As a nurse, you can help provide a space that promotes the patient's emotional, physical and spiritual well-being, as well as their comfort during this critical time.

Spatial planning :
- **Brightness:** Make sure the lighting in the room is soft and soothing, avoiding bright lights that could cause discomfort.
- **Layout:** Arrange the furniture to create an open, easily accessible space for the patient and visitors.

Comfortable furniture :
- **Comfortable bed:** Make sure the patient's bed is equipped with a comfortable mattress and cushions to promote restful sleep.

- **Chairs and rest areas:** Provide chairs and rest areas for relatives and visitors so that they can stay close to the patient.

Creating a soothing atmosphere :
- **Soft music:** Play soft, soothing music to create a serene atmosphere in the room.
- **Aromatherapy:** Use essential oils such as lavender or chamomile to bring a feeling of calm.

Personalising the Space :
- **Familiar objects:** If possible, place personal or family objects in the patient's room to create a familiar environment.
- **Photos and mementos:** Display meaningful photos and mementos to help the patient feel surrounded by loved ones.

Privacy and Confidentiality :
- **Curtains:** Use curtains or partitions to give patients and their families some privacy.
- **Respect for space:** Ensure that confidential discussions and intimate moments between patients and their families are respected.

Setting the Temperature :
- **Thermal comfort: Make sure the** room temperature is adapted to the patient's preferences, so that it is neither too hot nor too cold.
- **Blankets and cushions:** Have light blankets and extra cushions available to meet the patient's needs.

Avoiding Uncomfortable Stimuli :
- **Noise Reduction:** Minimise loud or disruptive noises that could disturb the calm of the environment.
- **Light control:** Use blackout curtains to control daylight and help the patient rest.

Creating a comfortable and soothing environment for palliative care patients can have a significant impact on their overall well-being. By considering the patient's individual preferences and providing an atmosphere that promotes comfort and tranquillity, you are helping to provide a space where the patient can feel surrounded by loving care during this delicate phase of life.

Planning for Comfort Care and Symptom Management

Planning comfort care and symptom management is a crucial step in palliative care for patients at the end of life. As a nurse, you play an essential role in developing a care plan that aims to maintain the patient's quality of life while effectively managing the symptoms associated with their condition.

Comprehensive Symptom Assessment :
- **Physical symptoms:** Identify and assess physical symptoms such as pain, dyspnoea, nausea and fatigue.
- **Psychological symptoms:** Explore psychological symptoms such as depression, anxiety and confusion.

Interdisciplinary collaboration :
- **Care Team:** Work with the medical team, mental health professionals and social workers to create a comprehensive care plan.
- **Communication:** Communicate regularly with other team members to ensure effective coordination of care.

Personalising the Care Plan :
- **Patient preferences:** Incorporate the patient's preferences and priorities into the care plan to ensure they receive care tailored to their needs.
- **Care Goals:** Identify the patient's care goals, whether they are to relieve pain, maintain mobility or promote inner peace.

Pain and Symptom Management :
- **Medication:** Plan for adequate pain management using appropriate medication and techniques.
- **Non-medicinal therapies:** Incorporate therapies such as relaxation, meditation and music therapy to manage symptoms.

Regular monitoring :
- **Ongoing assessment:** Regularly reassess the patient's symptoms and adjust the care plan in line with their progress.
- **Active listening:** Pay attention to the patient's signals about changing symptoms and needs.

Patient and Family Education :
- **Information on Symptoms:** Explain to the patient and family the possible symptoms and how to manage them.
- **Home management:** Provide instructions on how to manage symptoms at home and what to do if they worsen.

Documenting and communicating:
- **Medical records:** Carefully document the care plan, symptoms and interventions in the patient's medical record.
- **Transparent communication:** Share relevant information with the care team to ensure holistic care.

Planning for comfort care and symptom management requires a proactive and coordinated approach. By working with the care team, tailoring the plan to the patient's preferences and keeping an eye on how the situation is evolving, you help to ensure that the patient receives appropriate, high-quality care while maintaining a good quality of life during this delicate period.

Accompanying patients in their final moments

Empathic Presence and Emotional Support

Empathy and emotional support are essential aspects of palliative care for patients at the end of life. As a nurse, you play a key role in providing attentive listening, empathic understanding and emotional support to patients and their families during this sensitive period.

Establishing a Calm and Caring Presence :
- **Non-invasive approach:** Respect the patient's space while showing that you are available for any interaction.
- **Visual contact:** Make warm eye contact to express your care and commitment.

Active Listening and Empathic Understanding :
- **Listening without Judgement:** Let the patient express themselves freely without interrupting, judging or offering immediate solutions.
- **Validation of Emotions:** Express empathy by validating the patient's emotions and showing that you understand how they feel.

Emotional Support for Families :
- **Welcome Emotions:** Provide a space where families can openly express their concerns and emotions.
- **Sharing information:** Provide honest and understandable information to help families better understand the situation.

Offering moments of comfort:
- **Silent presence:** Be present in a silent way when the patient or family needs to think or reflect.
- **Emotional support:** Offer gentle physical contact, such as holding hands, if appropriate and desired.

Validation of experience :
- **Normalization:** Explain that the patient's emotions, concerns and experiences are normal in this context.
- **Listening without judging:** Avoid judging the patient's emotional reactions and make sure they feel safe to share them.

Meeting Spiritual and Emotional Needs :
- **Spiritual questions:** If the patient expresses spiritual questions, engage in open and respectful discussions.
- **Presence for Important Moments:** Be present for significant moments, such as end-of-life discussions or preparations for the funeral ceremony.

Practising Compassion in Action :
- **Helping with the Little Things:** Offer your help with everyday tasks that can relieve the patient and the family.
- **Anticipating needs:** Try to anticipate the emotional and practical needs of the patient and family before they express them.

The empathetic presence and emotional support you offer patients and their families are essential elements in creating an environment of trust, respect and caring. By actively listening, showing empathy and responding to emotional needs, you help to ease the emotional burden for everyone and support them sensitively during this delicate phase of life.

Relieving Anxiety and Physical Discomfort

Relieving anxiety and physical discomfort is a priority in palliative care for patients at the end of life. As a nurse, you have a crucial role to play in helping patients feel more comfortable emotionally and physically during this delicate period.

Assessment of Anxiety :
- **Observation:** Look out for signs of anxiety such as agitation, nervousness and sleep disturbance.
- **Communication:** Ask open-ended questions to understand the sources of the patient's anxiety.

Approaches to Relieving Anxiety :
- **Active listening:** Offer an attentive ear so that the patient can express his or her concerns and worries.
- **Relaxation techniques:** Teach techniques such as deep breathing, meditation and visualisation to reduce anxiety.

Physical Discomfort Management :
- **Pain:** Ensure that the pain management plan is adapted to the patient's needs and adjust it accordingly.
- **Nausea and vomiting:** Use anti-emetic medication and offer techniques such as acupressure to relieve these symptoms.

Reassuring Communication:
- **Clear information:** Provide honest information about the patient's situation and the measures taken to manage anxiety and discomfort.
- **Management options:** Involve the patient in decisions about methods of managing anxiety and discomfort.

Use of Complementary Therapies :
- **Massage therapy:** If appropriate, offer gentle massage sessions to relieve body tension and promote relaxation.
- **Art therapies:** Encourage the patient to take part in creative activities such as painting or music to reduce stress.

Interdisciplinary collaboration :
- **Teamwork:** Collaborate with doctors, psychologists and other health professionals to offer a comprehensive approach.
- **Social work:** If necessary, involve a social worker to offer extra support with anxieties and financial concerns.

Ongoing assessment :
- **Adjustments:** Monitor the effectiveness of interventions and adjust them if necessary to ensure patient comfort.
- **Patient feedback:** Listen carefully to how the patient reacts to different approaches to relief.

By relieving anxiety and physical discomfort, you help to improve a patient's quality of life at the end of life. Your ability to listen, to adjust care to individual needs and to collaborate with other healthcare professionals plays an essential role in providing compassionate care tailored to each patient.

Facilitating final communication between patients and their relatives

Facilitating final communication between the patient and their loved ones is a delicate but important task in palliative care for patients at the end of life. As a nurse, you can play a vital role in creating a space where patients and their loved ones can have meaningful conversations, express their feelings and share precious memories.

Creating a space conducive to communication :
- **Privacy:** Make sure the environment is quiet and private, providing a place where conversations can take place without interruption.
- **Discreet presence:** Be present if loved ones need your support, but make sure you don't interfere in their exchanges.

Encouraging Important Conversations:
- **Open discussion:** Encourage loved ones and the patient to discuss important issues such as end-of-life wishes and concerns freely.
- **Clarify misunderstandings:** If misunderstandings arise, act as a go-between to help clarify things.

Supporting Emotional Communication :
- **Emotional validations:** Show understanding and empathy for the emotions expressed by the patient and those close to them.
- **Expressing feelings:** Encourage everyone to share their feelings and memories without judgement.

Introducing Difficult Questions :
- **End of life:** If the patient wishes, facilitate discussions about the end of life, wishes regarding care and difficult decisions.
- **Funeral planning:** If appropriate, offer resources to help plan funeral arrangements.

Promoting the exchange of important messages:
- **Letters and messages:** Encourage patients and relatives to write letters or messages to express their thoughts and feelings.
- **Create Memories:** Make it easy to create tangible memories such as audio recordings or videos for loved ones.

Supporting patients in their communication objectives :
- • **Leading the conversation:** If the patient wishes, act as a mediator to help guide the conversation towards the subjects they wish to discuss.
- • **Allow time:** Be patient and allow time for the patient to express their feelings.

Respecting Spiritual Beliefs :
- • **Rituals and prayers:** If the patient and family wish, support the practice of meaningful rituals or prayers.
- • **Spiritual comfort:** Offer spiritual support if it corresponds to the beliefs of the patient and their family.

Facilitating the final communication between the patient and their loved ones requires deep sensitivity and understanding on the part of the nurse. By creating an open and caring space for conversations, encouraging the expression of feelings and supporting the individual needs of the patient and their family, you can help create precious moments of connection and meaningful farewell.

Ritual and Spirituality in Palliative Care

Integrating the patient's spiritual and religious beliefs
Integrating the patient's spiritual and religious beliefs is a crucial dimension of palliative care for patients at the end of life. As a nurse, you must respect and take into account the patient's personal beliefs in order to provide holistic support that meets their spiritual and emotional needs.

Respectful approach :
- • **Active listening:** Listen attentively to the patient when they share their spiritual and religious beliefs, without judgement.
- • **Sensitive questions:** If the patient is open to talking about it, ask open-ended questions to better understand their spirituality.

Coordination with Religious Personnel :
- • **Spiritual leaders:** If the patient wishes, facilitate a visit from a religious leader or spiritual adviser of their faith.
- • **Religious resources:** Provide religious resources such as sacred texts or specific prayers if the patient requests them.

Incorporation into Care :
- **Rituals and prayers:** If the patient wishes to have specific rituals or prayers, make sure they are respected as far as possible.
- **Food: Take** any dietary restrictions or religious preferences into account when planning meals.

Emotional and Spiritual Support :
- **Spiritual reassurance:** Offer your support by listening to the patient and sharing spiritual reflections where appropriate.
- **Prayer support:** If the patient wishes, you can take part in prayers or meditations.

Respect for Practices and Ceremonies :
- **Planning ceremonies:** If the patient expresses the wish for a specific ceremony, help to organise it in collaboration with the family and religious resources.
- **Privacy:** Ensure that patients can practise their faith in private if they so wish.

Adapting to Changing Needs :
- **Evolution of beliefs:** Be aware that a patient's spiritual beliefs may evolve depending on the medical and emotional situation.
- **Care adjustments:** Adapt care to the spiritual needs of patients throughout their end-of-life journey.

Cultural sensitivity :
- **Cultural context:** Be aware of the cultural practices associated with the patient's spiritual and religious beliefs.
- **Advice from the family:** If the family shares information about the patient's beliefs, take note of them and respect them.

Integrating patients' spiritual and religious beliefs into palliative care requires deep sensitivity and respect. By listening, offering appropriate spiritual support and collaborating with religious resources where necessary, you help to create a compassionate care environment that recognises and respects the spiritual dimension of the patient at the end of life.

Offering moments of reflection and prayer

Offering moments for reflection and prayer is an important way of integrating the spiritual dimension into palliative care for patients at the end of life. As a nurse, you can play a significant role in creating spaces and opportunities for patients and their loved ones to connect spiritually and find comfort.

Listening and Respect :
- **Patient preferences:** If the patient has expressed religious or spiritual preferences, respect them by offering time for reflection or prayer in line with their faith.
- **Respectful invitation:** Propose these moments delicately, leaving the patient and his or her family free to decide whether they wish to participate.

Creating a peaceful space:
- **Quiet environment:** Choose a quiet space where patients and their loved ones can gather in peace.
- **Symbolic elements:** If the patient wishes, add symbolic elements such as candles, religious icons or significant personal objects.

Facilitating reflection :
- **Gentle Guidance:** If the patient wishes, offer a short reflection or inspirational thoughts related to spirituality or the end of life.
- **Time to reflect:** Offer a time of silence to allow participants to meditate, reflect or pray in their own way.

Inclusion of Relatives :
- **Invitation to family and friends:** Encourage family and friends to join in these moments of reflection and prayer if they wish.
- **Sharing memories:** You can invite participants to share memories, thoughts or prayers in honour of the patient.

Respect for Diversity:
- **Cultural adaptation:** Be aware of cultural and religious diversity and ensure that moments of reflection respect these differences.
- **Inclusive approach:** If religious diversity is present, ensure that all participants feel comfortable and respected.

Spiritual Assistance :
- **Spiritual support:** If the patient wishes to have a religious leader or spiritual adviser present, coordinate their visit during these moments of reflection.
- **Respect for autonomy:** Make sure that patients and their families feel free to choose whether or not they want spiritual assistance during these times.

Offering moments of reflection and prayer can bring profound comfort to patients and their loved ones during the end-of-life period. By creating a space of serenity and respect, you enable participants to explore and nurture their spiritual dimension in a meaningful way, which can contribute to a sense of peace and connection at this delicate time.

Facilitating farewells and end-of-life rituals
Facilitating goodbyes and end-of-life rituals is a deeply meaningful task in palliative care for patients at the end of life. As a nurse, you can play a vital role in helping patients and their loved ones create memorable and meaningful moments that honour their journey and foster emotional connection.

Creating a Respectful Space :
- **Privacy:** Provide a private space where patients and their loved ones can meet in complete tranquillity.
- **Welcoming practices:** Respect the cultural and religious practices of patients and their families by adapting the space accordingly.

Facilitating personal farewells:
- **Quality time:** Encourage loved ones to spend quality time with the patient, sharing memories and expressing their feelings.
- **Last Words:** Create an environment where patients can say goodbye to their loved ones and share messages of love and affection.

Support for end-of-life rituals :
- **Religious rituals:** Facilitate the performance of rituals specific to the patient's faith, such as prayers, blessings or symbolic practices.
- **Creating rituals:** If the patient and their family wish, suggest personalised rituals to mark the transition.

Coordination with religious leaders:
- **Spiritual visits:** If the patient wishes to have a religious leader present, coordinate their visit to facilitate rituals and prayers.
- **Active participation:** Encourage the patient and those close to them to take an active part in the rituals according to their beliefs.

Documentation and Memorabilia :
- **Photos and videos: With** the permission of the patient and family, document special moments to create tangible memories.

117

- **Logbook:** Give your loved ones the chance to keep a logbook of shared moments and goodbyes.

Emotional Support :

- **Empathic listening:** Be attentive to the emotional needs of the patient and those close to them at this delicate time.
- **Accompaniment:** Offer a compassionate presence when needed, listening to emotions and concerns.

Respect for time and privacy:

- **Leave control:** Respect the way in which the patient and their family wish to organise the farewell, leaving them in control of the process.
- **Personalised   time:** Allow each family to decide when and how they wish to participate in these end-of-life moments.

Facilitating farewells and end-of-life rituals can create precious and meaningful memories for patients and their loved ones. Your role is to offer emotional and practical support while respecting everyone's beliefs and practices. By facilitating these moments of connection and farewell, you help to make the end-of-life period smoother and more memorable for everyone involved.

Chapter 9:
Teamwork in Palliative Care

Collaboration between nurses, doctors and other professionals

Roles and responsibilities of nurses

Nurses play an essential role in providing high-quality palliative care for patients at the end of life. Their commitment, clinical expertise and compassion help to create a supportive environment that meets the physical, emotional and spiritual needs of patients and their families. Here is an exploration of the key roles and responsibilities of nurses:

Full Assessment :
- **Medical history:** Gathering the patient's complete medical history to understand their current condition and medical history.
- **Symptom Assessment:** In-depth assessment of the patient's symptoms and adaptation of care plans as the condition evolves.

Custom Planning :
- **Care Plan:** Developing individualised care plans in collaboration with the medical team and the patient's relatives.
- **Symptom management:** Using pharmacological and non-pharmacological approaches to manage pain and symptoms.

Emotional Support :
- **Empathetic listening:** Offering patients and their families an attentive ear, creating a space for them to express their emotions and concerns.
- **Spiritual support:** Recognising the importance of the spiritual dimension and offering support adapted to the patient's spirituality.

Sensitive Communication :
- **Open Dialogue:** Facilitating honest discussions about end of life, treatment options and goals of care.

- **Comprehensible information:** sensitively explaining complex medical information in a way that patients and their families can understand.

Interdisciplinary coordination :

- **Collaboration:** Working closely with doctors, social workers, spiritual advisers and other members of the care team.
- **Team meetings:** Participating in team meetings to discuss care plans, changes in the patient's condition and approaches to be taken.

Care for relatives :

- **Family Education:** Providing information and education to families about palliative care, treatments and options.
- **Emotional support:** Helping loved ones to cope with the emotions associated with the end of life and to understand their role in care.

Documenting Care :

- **Medical records:** Maintaining accurate and complete records of the care provided, including care decisions taken in collaboration with the patient and their family.
- **Status reports:** Provide regular reports on the patient's condition to the medical team and other healthcare professionals.

Self-care and stress management :

- **Self-care:** Recognising the importance of taking care of yourself to prevent burnout.
- **Stress management:** Developing strategies for managing the emotional stress associated with palliative care.

As a nurse, you embody compassion and understanding for patients and their families during this sensitive time. Your role extends beyond physical care to include emotional support, open communication and interdisciplinary teamwork. By providing holistic care that respects the dignity and wishes of the patient, you create as comfortable and meaningful an end-of-life experience as possible.

The Importance of Communication with Doctors

Effective communication between nurses and doctors is crucial to ensuring consistent, high-quality, patient-centred care. Close collaboration between these two professions contributes to informed decision-making, coordinated care plans and overall patient and family satisfaction. This is why communication with physicians is of paramount importance in palliative care:

Co-Creation of Care Plans :
- **Information exchange:** Nurses provide valuable information about symptoms, patient reactions and changes in health status that help doctors make informed treatment decisions.
- **Holistic approach:** Nurses can provide information about the patient's emotional, psychological and spiritual needs, contributing to more comprehensive care plans.

Real-time adjustments :
- **Patient reactions:** The nurses observe the patient's reactions to treatments and medicines and pass this information on to the doctors for rapid adjustments.
- **Ongoing assessment:** Open communication allows doctors to obtain regular updates on the patient's condition, which is essential for adapting care as the condition evolves.

Shared decision-making :
- **Inclusion of Relatives:** Nurses can provide perspectives from the patient's relatives, which contributes to shared decision-making centred on the patient's wishes.
- **Treatment options:** Doctors and nurses can work together to discuss different treatment options, taking into account the benefits, risks and preferences of the patient.

Improving the quality of care :
- **Early detection:** Proactive communication between nurses and doctors enables early detection of complications or emerging symptoms, which can prevent more serious problems.
- **Regular monitoring:** Doctors can request regular reports from nurses to monitor the patient's response to treatment and adapt plans accordingly.

Emotional Support for Doctors:
- **Emotional burden:** Nurses can provide emotional support to doctors by helping them to understand the impact of end-of-life decisions on patients and their families.
- **Collaborative consultation:** Nurses can share their expertise in symptom management and sensitive communication to help doctors tackle difficult subjects.

Open and regular communication between nurses and doctors promotes mutual understanding, optimal coordination and patient-centred care. This collaboration enhances the quality of care offered to patients at the end of life and creates an environment where medical, emotional and spiritual needs are addressed holistically.

Working with therapists, social workers and others

Interdisciplinary collaboration is at the heart of quality palliative care. By working as a team with other healthcare professionals such as therapists, social workers and other members of the care team, nurses can offer a holistic approach that meets the complex needs of patients at the end of life. Here's why working with these professionals is essential:

Global Approach to the Patient :
- **Specialist expertise:** Therapists, such as palliative care counsellors, psychologists and spiritual advisors, provide their expertise to help patients and their families deal with the emotional, psychological and spiritual aspects of the end of life.
- **Social support:** Social workers help to identify the resources and social support needed to meet the practical and emotional needs of patients and their families.

Collaborative Decision Making :
- **Taking Perspectives into Account:** Different healthcare professionals bring unique perspectives to care decisions, integrating medical, psychological, social and spiritual aspects.
- **Care Objectives:** Working together, we can define care objectives that are tailored to the patient's individual needs, taking into account all aspects of their situation.

Symptom Management :
- **Multidisciplinary approach:** The management of complex symptoms can benefit from a multidisciplinary approach, where nurses collaborate with doctors and therapists to find the best solutions.
- **Integrated Care Plans:** By working together, professionals can develop integrated care plans that take into account pain management, psychological symptoms and emotional needs.

Emotional Support :
- **Teamwork:** Collaboration with therapists and social workers enables more comprehensive emotional support to be provided to patients and their families, drawing on different areas of expertise.
- **Coordination of resources:** Social workers help coordinate the resources and services needed to meet housing, financial and social support needs.

Continuity of care :
- **Smooth transitions:** Collaboration facilitates transitions between different levels of care, such as from hospital to home care or hospice.
- **Coordinated   follow-up:** Professionals work together to ensure consistent and regular follow-up, guaranteeing that the patient's needs are continually assessed.

By collaborating with therapists, social workers and other members of the care team, nurses offer a holistic approach that addresses the complex needs of patients at the end of life. This collaboration enhances the quality of care, improves symptom management and supports patients and their families through all aspects of their end-of-life journey.

Role of the Social Worker and Spirituality Advisor

Emotional, Psychological and Practical Support for Families
Supporting the families of palliative care patients is an essential part of palliative care nursing practice. Families face a variety of emotions, psychological challenges and practical needs during this delicate time. Nurses play a crucial role in providing emotional, psychological and practical support to help them through this journey.

Emotional Support :
- **Active listening:** Listen carefully to your loved ones and encourage them to express their feelings, fears and concerns.
- **Validating emotions:** Validate families' emotions, recognising that every reaction is legitimate in this difficult situation.

- **Empathy:** Show empathy by putting yourself in their shoes, understanding their pain and expressing your understanding.

Psychological support :
- **Advice:** Offer advice and information to help families understand what to expect during the end-of-life process.
- **Stress Management:** Provide stress management techniques and strategies for dealing with the intense emotions associated with the situation.
- **Referral to therapists:** Refer families to palliative care counsellors, psychologists or mental health professionals for more specialist support.

Practical Support :
- **Logistical organisation:** Help families organise care, coordinate visiting schedules and understand medical procedures.
- **Coordinating resources:** Inform families about available resources, such as home services, social supports and support groups.
- **Material assistance:** Offer advice on practical matters such as funeral arrangements, legal documents and logistical preparations.

Spiritual support :
- **Respect for beliefs:** Respect families' spiritual and religious beliefs by providing spiritual support tailored to their needs.
- **Facilitating rituals:** If the family wishes, facilitate the creation of spaces for prayer, meditation or other spiritual rituals.

Education :
- **Understanding Symptoms:** Educating families about the symptoms the patient may experience at the end of life can reduce anxiety and uncertainty.
- **End-of-life process:** Explain the physical, emotional and psychological changes that can occur during the end-of-life process, so that families are better prepared.

Preserving Dignity:
- **Respect for confidentiality:** Ensure that sensitive information about patients and their families is treated with the utmost discretion.
- **Respectful communication:** Communicate with families with sensitivity, taking into account their values, preferences and level of understanding.

Emotional, psychological and practical support for families is an essential part of the holistic approach to palliative care. By offering compassionate support and responding to the varied needs of families, nurses help to create an environment where patients and their families feel cared for and supported throughout their end-of-life journey.

Integrating the Spiritual Dimension into Palliative Care

Spirituality in palliative care is a holistic approach that recognises the importance of spirituality for patients and their families at the end of life. Spirituality can be a source of comfort, meaning and healing, and nurses play an essential role in meeting patients' spiritual needs and creating an environment conducive to spiritual reflection and growth.

Listening and exploring :
- **Openness to Discussion:** Create a space where patients and their families feel comfortable discussing spiritual and religious topics.
- **Sensitive questioning:** Ask open-ended questions to encourage patients to explore their spirituality, beliefs and concerns.

Respect for beliefs :
- **Diversity:** Be aware of the diversity of spiritual and religious beliefs and respect individual convictions.
- **Beliefs and practices:** Find out about the patient's specific spiritual beliefs and practices so that you can respond appropriately to their needs.

Spiritual support :
- **Counselling and support:** Offer spiritual counselling and support according to the patient's needs and requests, working with spiritual advisers if necessary.
- **Rituals and prayers:** Facilitate participation in religious rituals, prayers or moments of meditation, if the patient so wishes.

Finding meaning :
- **Reflecting on life:** Encourage patients to reflect on the meaning of their lives, to find comfort in their beliefs and to make peace with their spiritual values.
- **Acceptance:** Help patients find a space to accept the end of life through a spiritual perspective that can bring a sense of serenity.

125

Family support :
- **Family and Spirituality:** Provide spiritual support to the patient's family at the end of life, recognising that spirituality can be important to them too.
- **Spiritual meetings:** Organise family get-togethers or times of prayer if the family wishes, to encourage spiritual connection.

Facilitating Healing :
- **Inner healing:** Help patients find ways to heal on a spiritual level by reconciling with themselves, others and their beliefs.
- **Creative expression:** Encourage patients to use creative expression, such as writing, art or music, to explore their emotions and spirituality.

Integrating the spiritual dimension into palliative care offers a comprehensive approach that recognises and respects the spirituality of patients and their families. By addressing these issues with sensitivity and providing appropriate support, nurses help to create a deeper, more meaningful end-of-life experience that is aligned with the patient's personal beliefs and values.

Coordination of Resources and External Aid

Co-ordinating resources and outside help is an essential part of nurses' role in ensuring that patients and their families receive the support they need during this difficult time. By working closely with other health and social care professionals and support organisations, nurses ensure that patients have access to a full range of resources to meet their diverse needs.

Needs Assessment :
- **Identify Needs:** Discuss with patients and their families what their specific needs are in terms of practical, emotional, financial and spiritual support.
- **Assess Available Resources:** Identify existing resources in the community, such as home care programmes, support groups and counselling services.

Coordination of Services :
- **Referrals:** Refer patients to specific services according to their needs, such as therapists, social workers, spiritual counsellors and support groups.

- **Liaison with Medical Services:** Coordinate care with doctors, specialists and other health professionals involved in the patient's follow-up.

Psychosocial support :
- **Emotional Support:** Refer patients and families to palliative care counsellors, psychologists or social workers for more specialised emotional support.
- **Support Groups:** Inform patients and families about local support groups where they can connect with others going through similar situations.

Material Assistance :
- **Financial assistance:** Identify the financial resources available to help patients and families meet medical costs and material needs.
- **Aides à Domicile:** Organise access to home help services to assist patients with their daily activities.

Home Care Coordination :
- **Palliative Home Care Services:** Work with home care services to ensure patients receive quality care in the comfort of their own home.
- **Carer training:** Provide training for family members and carers on how to provide basic care at home.

Facilitating access to resources :
- **Logistical organisation:** Help patients and their families organise medical appointments, home visits and other logistical aspects of care.
- **Ongoing monitoring:** Ensure that patients and families have ongoing access to the services and resources they need.

By coordinating resources and facilitating access to outside help, nurses help to ease the burden on patients and their families during this delicate period. By providing well-coordinated practical, emotional and social support, nurses ensure that patients can focus on their well-being and quality of life at the end of life.

The Importance of Coordination for Optimal Care

Interdisciplinary Planning and Communication
Interdisciplinary planning and communication are key elements of quality palliative care. Nurses work closely with other healthcare professionals to develop comprehensive and coordinated care plans that meet the complex needs of patients at the end of life. This interdisciplinary approach ensures holistic and coherent care that aims to optimise the patient's quality of life.

Care Planning :
- **Team meetings:** Participate in interdisciplinary team meetings to discuss patient needs, share information and develop integrated care plans.
- **Specialist collaboration:** Consult and collaborate with doctors, therapists, social workers and other professionals to develop a comprehensive care plan.

Transparent communication :
- **Information Sharing:** Share relevant information about the patient's condition, symptoms, care goals and preferences with other team members.
- **Exchange of Expertise:** Benefit from the unique expertise of each professional to contribute to informed decision-making and care planning.

Cooperation for Symptoms :
- **Symptom management:** Work with doctors and specialists to develop symptom management plans, combining pharmacological and non-pharmacological approaches.
- **Real-time adjustments:** Communicate regularly to adjust treatment plans in line with changes in the patient's condition.

Care objectives :
- **Coordination of objectives: Ensure** that care objectives are aligned between team members, taking into account the patient's wishes and values.
- **Plan development:** Integrate the perspectives of each professional in the development of personalised care plans that meet the patient's multiple needs.

Anticipating needs :
- **Short- and long-term preparation:** Work with team members to anticipate the future needs of the patient and their family, putting plans in place to meet those needs.
- **Transition Planning:** Coordinate the transition between different levels of care, such as hospital, home care or hospice.

Continuity of care :
- **Smooth transitions:** Make sure that information on care plans and objectives is passed on smoothly during transitions between healthcare professionals.
- **Regular monitoring:** Ensure ongoing monitoring by communicating regularly with other team members to assess progress and make adjustments if necessary.

Interdisciplinary planning and communication are essential pillars of effective and consistent palliative care. By working as a team with other healthcare professionals, nurses ensure that each patient benefits from a comprehensive, personalised and holistic care plan that meets their individual needs and preferences.

Regular monitoring of patient progress and needs

Regular monitoring of a patient's progress and needs throughout their palliative care journey is crucial to ensuring high quality and appropriate care. Nurses play an essential role in carefully monitoring the patient's condition, adjusting care plans accordingly and responding to changing needs throughout this delicate period.

Ongoing assessment :
- **Regular assessment:** Carry out regular assessments of the patient's physical, emotional and psychological state to detect changes and emerging needs.
- **Symptoms and Comfort:** Closely monitor patient symptoms such as pain, dyspnoea and nausea, adjusting treatment plans as necessary.

Communication with the Team :
- **Information transfer:** Share observations and updates with other members of the interdisciplinary team for a coordinated approach.

- **Collaborative Care:** Work closely with doctors, therapists and other professionals to adjust care plans and goals to meet changing needs.

Making Informed Decisions :

- **Informing Decisions:** Provide the patient and family with up-to-date information on the patient's condition to help them make informed decisions.
- **Treatment options:** Discuss possible treatment options based on the evolving medical situation and the patient's preferences.

Short-term care planning :

- **Rapid adaptations:** Be ready to make immediate adjustments to care plans in response to urgent needs or new situations.
- **Symptom Management:** Respond quickly to emerging symptoms by adjusting medication, therapies and non-pharmacological approaches.

Communication with the Patient and Family :

- **Regular reporting:** Keep the patient and family informed of progress and care plans, helping them to understand changes.
- **Answers to Questions:** Answer the questions and concerns of patients and their families, providing clear and appropriate information.

Anticipating future needs :

- **Anticipate changes:** Consider future needs based on the patient's condition and observed trends, and be prepared to adjust plans accordingly.
- **Collaboration in Forecasting:** Work with team members to anticipate potential needs and develop long-term support plans.

Regular monitoring of the patient's progress and needs ensures that palliative care remains appropriate and responsive to the changes that occur during the end-of-life period. Nurses play a vital role by carefully monitoring the patient's condition, communicating effectively with the interdisciplinary team and providing ongoing coordination to ensure that the patient receives the most appropriate care at every stage of their journey.

Managing Care Transitions to Ensure Continuity

Managing transitions of care is a crucial component of palliative care, as patients may move through different levels of care and care settings throughout their journey. Nurses play an essential role in planning and coordinating transitions to ensure effective continuity of care, minimising disruption for patients and their families.

Early planning :
- **Early discussion:** Start discussing potential transitions with the patient and family as soon as possible, explaining the different care options and the benefits of each transition.
- **Anticipating needs:** Anticipate the patient's future needs in terms of care and environment, so you can plan accordingly.

Communication Claire :
- **Full information:** Provide full information on transitions, including reasons for the transition, benefits, implications and expected changes.
- **Answering Questions:** Be prepared to answer any questions the patient and family may have about the transition, providing clear and reassuring answers.

Care Coordination :
- **Smooth transfer:** Work closely with healthcare professionals in the care facilities to which the patient is transferred, ensuring that information and care plans are shared transparently.
- **Liaising with the team:** Communicate with the interdisciplinary team to ensure that all aspects of the patient's care are taken into account during the transition.

Preparing the Patient and Family :
- **Education:** Provide information about upcoming care, new care teams and services available at the new destination.
- **Realistic expectations:** Help the patient and family to have realistic expectations of the new care situation and to prepare themselves emotionally.

Continuity of Care Objectives :
- **Transfer of objectives:** Ensure that the care objectives previously defined are maintained and adapted during the transition.

- **Long-term   planning:** Work with the team to develop a long-term care plan that takes into account possible future transitions.

Follow-up after the transition :

- **Transition check: Make sure** that the transition has gone smoothly and that the patient has been welcomed and cared for appropriately.
- **Regular monitoring:** Continue to monitor the patient's condition and adjust care plans as necessary, even after transition.

Successfully managing transitions of care is essential to ensuring continuity of high quality palliative care and minimising disruption for patients and their families. By effectively planning, communicating and coordinating transitions, nurses ensure that patients continue to receive consistent and appropriate care, wherever they are in their end-of-life journey.

Chapter 10:
Self-care for nurses

Managing Stress and Burnout

Recognising the signs of stress and burn-out

The role of a nurse is both rewarding and demanding. Working with patients at the end of life and their families can be emotionally and physically taxing. It is crucial for nurses to recognise the signs of stress and burn-out so that they can take steps to preserve their mental, emotional and physical well-being.

Signs of stress :
- **Persistent fatigue:** If you feel constantly exhausted, even after adequate rest, this could be a sign of stress.
- **Increased irritability:** A drop in your tolerance threshold and increased irritability can be indicators of stress.
- **Difficulty concentrating:** If you find it hard to concentrate on your tasks or make decisions, this may be the result of stress.
- **Insomnia or disturbed sleep:** Frequent sleep problems, such as insomnia or frequent waking, can be linked to stress.

Signs of burn-out :
- **Emotional detachment:** If you feel emotionally exhausted and detached from your patients and your work, this may indicate burn-out.
- **Cynicism and dehumanisation:** Cynicism towards patients or colleagues and dehumanisation of patients are classic signs of burn-out.
- **Decreased job satisfaction:** When you lose your sense of satisfaction and fulfilment at work, it can be a sign of burn-out.
- **Decreased energy:** If even simple tasks seem overwhelming and exhausting, this may be linked to burn-out.

Physical symptoms :
- **Frequent headaches :** Frequent headaches and body aches can be physical manifestations of stress and burn-out.
- **Digestive problems:** Gastrointestinal problems, such as stomach upsets and digestive problems, can be exacerbated by stress.
- **Weak immune system:** Chronic stress can weaken your immune system, making you more vulnerable to infection.

Behavioural changes :
- **Social withdrawal:** If you avoid social interaction and prefer isolation, this may be a sign of stress.
- **Use of Negative Coping Mechanisms :** Excessive use of alcohol, tobacco or substances to cope with stress is a warning sign.
- **Increased procrastination:** If you find it difficult to complete your professional and personal tasks, this may be the result of stress.

It is essential to recognise these signs as soon as they appear and to take steps to prevent stress and burn-out. Taking care of your emotional and physical well-being is crucial if you are to continue to provide quality care to palliative care patients. Don't hesitate to seek professional support, implement self-care strategies and seek resources to manage stress and maintain your balance.

Everyday Stress Management Techniques
Stress management is essential to maintaining your well-being as a nurse. Here are some practical techniques you can incorporate into your daily routine to reduce stress and promote your mental and emotional health.

1. Mindfulness practice :
Mindfulness involves focusing fully on the present moment, paying attention to your sensations, thoughts and emotions without judging them. This can help reduce stress by helping you to stay calm and centred in difficult situations.

2. Deep Breathing and Relaxation :
Take a few moments each day to practise deep breathing and relaxation exercises. These techniques can help reduce physical and mental tension, giving you a moment of peace.

3. Regular physical exercise :

Exercise is an excellent way of reducing stress by releasing endorphins, mood-enhancing chemicals. Find a physical activity that you enjoy and try to fit it into your schedule on a regular basis.

4. Work-life balance :

It's important to define clear boundaries between work and personal life. Give yourself time for your hobbies, your favourite activities and your family, to recharge your batteries and reduce work-related stress.

5. Relaxation practices :

Explore different relaxation practices, such as yoga, meditation and stretching. These activities can help reduce muscle tension and calm the mind.

6. Time for You :

Give yourself regular time to relax and recharge. Reading, listening to music, spending time in nature or simply resting can help relieve stress.

7. Social support :

Maintain positive social relationships with colleagues, friends and family. Sharing your experiences and feelings can help ease the burden of stress.

8. Time Management :

Organise your time effectively by drawing up task lists and prioritising important activities. This can reduce the stress associated with work overload and managing multiple responsibilities.

9. Creative Practices :

Get involved in creative activities such as painting, writing, music or crafts. These activities can act as a calming escape.

10. Seeking Professional Support :

If the stress becomes overwhelming, consider consulting a mental health professional or joining support groups. Talking about your challenges and getting advice can make a big difference.

11. Sleep Hygiene :

Make sure you maintain proper sleep hygiene by following a regular sleep routine and creating an environment conducive to rest.

By incorporating these stress management techniques into your daily routine, you can strengthen your emotional resilience and your ability to cope with the challenges of palliative care.

Maintaining your own well-being will enable you to continue to provide high quality, caring care to patients and their families.

Importance of Work-Life Balance
Work-life balance is essential for nurses. It is a vital practice that helps maintain the mental, emotional and physical health of healthcare professionals while ensuring the delivery of high quality care. Here's why work-life balance is so important in the context of palliative care:

1. Preventing burn-out :
Work-life balance helps prevent burn-out, which can develop when professional stress overwhelms your resources for coping. Working in palliative care is emotionally demanding, and taking regular breaks helps to recharge your energies.

2. Maintaining the quality of care :
When you take care of yourself, you're in better condition to take care of others. A healthy balance enables you to offer high-quality, attentive care, because you are more alert, focused and emotionally present.

3. Strengthening resilience :
A healthy balance helps to strengthen your emotional resilience, i.e. your ability to cope with challenges and stresses without becoming exhausted. You'll be better prepared to handle the difficult situations that naturally arise in palliative care.

4. Preserving personal relationships :
Work-life balance allows you to devote time to your personal relationships and your family. These social connections provide essential emotional support and help maintain your well-being.

5. Preventing emotional exhaustion :
When you over-invest professionally to the detriment of your personal life, you run the risk of emotional exhaustion. Taking time for yourself helps you maintain your emotional balance.

6. Increased productivity :
A healthy balance promotes better time management and greater efficiency in your work. You'll be more productive when you're well rested and take regular breaks.

7. Stress Reduction :
A work-life balance reduces stress levels, which has a positive impact on your overall health and your ability to manage the challenges of work.

8. Self-care and well-being :

Taking care of yourself is an act of self-compassion. By paying attention to your physical, emotional and mental well-being, you create an environment conducive to your own health and happiness.

Work-life balance not only benefits you as a nurse, it also contributes to the quality of care you provide. By investing in your own well-being, you create a virtuous circle where your mental and emotional health is reflected in your interactions with patients and their families, promoting a more positive care experience for all.

Personal Care Techniques to Preserve Mental Health

Relaxation and Mindfulness Practices

Relaxation and mindfulness practices are powerful tools for nurses, as they can help reduce stress, promote emotional resilience and maintain psychological balance. Incorporating these practices into your daily routine can help improve your overall wellbeing and your ability to provide high quality care. Here are some practices you might consider:

1. Mindfulness meditation :

Mindfulness meditation involves paying deliberate attention to the present moment, without judgement. You can sit comfortably, close your eyes and concentrate on your breathing, letting your thoughts pass without becoming attached to them.

2. Yoga :

Yoga combines gentle physical movement with concentrated attention to the breath. It can improve flexibility, reduce muscular tension and encourage a state of inner calm.

3. Breathing exercises :

Practise deep breathing exercises regularly. Take slow, deep breaths, inhaling through your nose and exhaling through your mouth. This can help calm the nervous system and reduce stress.

4. Mindfulness Walking :
When you walk, concentrate on the sensations of your feet touching the ground, the movement of your body and the environment around you. Walking mindfully can be calming and help you reconnect with the present moment.

5. Journaling :
Take a few minutes each day to write in a diary. This can include reflections on your emotions, experiences and thoughts. Journaling can be a **method of emotional release.**

6. Creative Practices :
Get involved in creative activities such as painting, writing, music or drawing. These activities allow you to channel your emotions and give you space to express yourself.

7. Conscious Musical Listening :
Sit comfortably and listen to music, concentrating solely on the sounds. Let yourself be absorbed by the music without being distracted by other thoughts.

8. Guided Viewing :
Use guided visualisation recordings to transport you mentally to peaceful, relaxing environments. This can help calm your mind and reduce stress.

9. Silent Time :
Create moments of silence in your day, when you simply allow yourself to be present and attentive, without distractions or worries.

10. Break times :
Take short breaks throughout the day to concentrate on your breathing and relax, even if only for a few minutes.

Experimenting with different relaxation and mindfulness practices will help you find the ones that work best for you. By making them a regular part of your routine, you can build emotional resilience, reduce stress and maintain a state of well-being that will help you provide optimal care to palliative care patients.

Maintaining healthy personal relationships
Maintaining healthy personal relationships is of paramount importance to nurses. The emotional challenges and demanding nature of your work further emphasise the need to cultivate strong bonds with those closest to you. These relationships can serve as a valuable resource to support you throughout your

138

career. Here are some tips for maintaining healthy personal relationships:

1. Open Communication :
Communicate openly and honestly with those closest to you. Share your experiences at work, your emotions and your needs. This can promote mutual understanding and support.

2. Quality time :
Make quality time for your loved ones. Avoid getting so caught up in the demands of work that you neglect precious time with your family and friends.

3. Set Limits :
Establish clear boundaries between your professional and personal life. Learn to say no when you need time for yourself or your loved ones.

4. Active listening :
When you spend time with your loved ones, practise active listening. Give them your full attention and express your interest in what they have to say.

5. Balance between responsibilities :
Find a balance between your responsibilities at work and your family and social responsibilities. Identify the times when you can be fully present with your loved ones.

6. Sharing Joy :
Don't just share the challenges of your job, but also the positive moments and successes. Celebrate your successes with those closest to you.

7. Mutual support :
Encourage an environment of mutual support. People close to you can be a source of comfort and encouragement **when you need to talk about your work.**

8. Respect everyone's needs:
Understand that each person has different needs and expectations in terms of time, space and attention. Respect these differences and adapt accordingly.

9. Integrating Relatives into Your Experience :
Whenever possible, share certain parts of your professional experience with those close to you. This can help them to better understand your role and offer you appropriate support.

10. Prioritise Quality Time:
Rather than quantifying the amount of time you spend with your loved ones, focus on the quality of that time. Even short

moments of meaningful connection can strengthen your relationships.

Cultivating healthy personal relationships helps create a strong support network that can help you manage the emotional challenges associated with your work in palliative care. Remember that sharing your experiences and emotions with those close to you can not only ease the emotional burden, but also strengthen your bonds and promote your own well-being.

Promoting an Active and Balanced Lifestyle
Encouraging an active and balanced lifestyle is crucial for nurses. The demanding pace of your work can make it difficult to prioritise your own health and wellbeing, but it's an essential part of maintaining your emotional and physical resilience. Here are some strategies for incorporating an active and balanced lifestyle into your daily routine:

1. Physical Activity Planning :
Build regular physical activity into your schedule. Whether it's a session at the gym, a walk, cycling or yoga, regular exercise can boost your energy and physical stamina.
2. Restorative walks :
If possible, take short walks during your breaks. Walking can be an excellent way to relax, reduce stress and improve circulation.
3. **Balanced diet :**
Opt for a balanced, nutritious diet. Avoid irregular diets and opt for a variety of foods that provide the nutrients you need to support your body.
4. Hydration :
Drink enough water throughout the day to keep hydrated. This can help maintain your energy and concentration.
5. Sleep Management :
Make sure you get quality sleep. Establish a regular sleep routine to ensure you get enough rest to recover.
6. Stress management :
Incorporate stress management techniques such as meditation, deep breathing and mindfulness to maintain emotional and mental balance.
7. Time for You :
Give yourself time for activities you enjoy outside work. This can include hobbies, pastimes or simply time to rest and relax.

8. Limits on overtime :
Avoid working excessive overtime. Prioritise a balance between work and rest.

9. Disconnection time :
When you're not at work, take the time to disconnect from screens and electronic devices. This will help you relax and improve the quality of your sleep.

10. Self-care :
Cultivate an attitude of self-care towards yourself. Listen to your physical, emotional and mental needs and respond appropriately.

Promoting an active and balanced lifestyle will help you maintain your vitality and resilience as a nurse. By taking care of your own health, you'll be better equipped to provide strong support to patients and their families. Remember that your wellbeing is fundamental to the quality of care you provide.

Continuing Education and Professional Development

The importance of training and updating knowledge
In the field of palliative care, continuing education and updating your knowledge are key to maintaining your professional competence and providing high-quality care. As palliative care evolves in response to medical advances, psychosocial approaches and changing patient needs, it is crucial to stay informed and well prepared. This is why training and updating knowledge are essential:

1. Evolution of practices :
The field of palliative care is constantly evolving, with new approaches, protocols and techniques emerging regularly. By taking part in training courses, you can learn the latest methods of pain management, psychological support and communication.

2. Improving the quality of care :
Ongoing training will enable you to improve the quality of care you provide to patients and their families. You will be better equipped to meet their changing needs and provide care based on current best practice.

3. Adapting to new challenges :
Training helps you to adapt to the new challenges and complexities that can arise in palliative care. For example, technological innovations or medical discoveries may require you to update your skills.

4. Building trust :
By being well-informed and competent, you will gain confidence in your professional skills. This will enable you to tackle difficult situations with confidence.

5. Encouraging innovation :
Continuing education encourages innovation. By learning new approaches and exploring different perspectives, you may discover innovative ways to improve the care you provide.

6. Maintaining relevance :
Continuing education keeps you up to date with the latest trends and advances in the field. This helps you stay relevant as a healthcare professional.

7. Personal development :
Training is not just limited to technical skills. It can also include aspects of personal development, such as stress management, effective communication and empathy.

8. Risk Reduction :
Proper training helps to reduce medical errors and prevent potentially dangerous situations for patients.

9. Commitment to Ethics :
Continuing education can include discussions on ethics and ethical dilemmas in palliative care. This will help you to navigate complex situations ethically.

10. Respect for Patients and Families :
By engaging in continuing education, you demonstrate your commitment to providing quality care to patients and families, which builds their confidence in you as a healthcare professional.

Taking part in regular training, conferences and workshops will ensure that you are at the cutting edge of the field of palliative care. It also demonstrates your dedication to your patients and your commitment to providing the best possible care in an ever-changing environment.

Participate in Support Groups and Supervisions

Participation in support groups and supervision is an effective way for nurses to look after their emotional well-being, connect with their peers and benefit from a space where they can share their experiences, challenges and successes. These forums provide essential support and promote personal and professional development. Here's why participating in support groups and supervision is important:

1. Sharing Experiences :
Support groups and supervisions provide a space to share your experiences, emotions and concerns with other professionals who understand the specific challenges of palliative care.

2. Validation and Support :
These groups allow you to feel validated and supported in your emotions. Other members can offer valuable insights, advice and encouragement.

3. Reduction of Insulation :
Working in palliative care can sometimes be emotionally isolating. Participating in support groups connects you with people who are going through similar experiences, which can reduce this feeling of isolation.

4. Personal development :
Reflection and discussion within these groups can encourage your personal and professional development. You can learn new strategies for dealing with challenges and improving your skills.

5. Learning from Others :
Hearing about other members' experiences can provide you with ideas and approaches that you may not have considered. This can enrich your care toolbox.

6. Emotional Relaxation :
Taking part in support groups and supervision provides a safe space to express your emotions and concerns, which can ease the emotional burden.

7. Burn-out prevention :
The support and advice you receive in these groups can help prevent burn-out by helping you to manage the stress and challenges associated with your work.

8. Reflective feedback :
Supervision sessions provide an opportunity to reflect on your interactions with patients and discuss difficult situations. This can strengthen your communication and decision-making skills.

9. Strengthening Compassion :
Listening to the stories and experiences of others can strengthen your ability to feel compassion for patients and their families.

10. Building Professional Relationships :
These groups can be an opportunity to build strong professional relationships with your peers, which can provide you with a long-term support network.

Participating in support groups and supervision can be a valuable resource for nurses. It can help you stay connected to your passion for caring, develop emotional resilience and maintain a healthy emotional and professional balance.

Career development: opportunities for specialisation and advancement
The field of palliative care offers many career development opportunities for nurses who wish to deepen their knowledge, develop their skills and take on leadership positions. These opportunities for specialisation and advancement can not only enhance your career, but also strengthen your impact as a healthcare professional. Here are some options to consider:

1. Specialisation in Advanced Palliative Care :
Some nurses choose to specialise further by taking advanced training courses in palliative care. These programmes deepen your knowledge and skills in specific areas such as complex pain management, advanced symptoms and paediatric palliative care.

2. Palliative Care Manager :
For those interested in leadership, becoming a palliative care manager is an option. You will be responsible for coordinating palliative care teams, managing resources and overseeing **day-to-day** operations.

3. Education and training :
If you have a passion for teaching, you could consider becoming a palliative care trainer or teacher. You can help train the next generation of specialist palliative care nurses.

4. Consultation and advice :
Some nurses choose to become consultants or advisers in healthcare establishments, sharing their expertise to improve palliative care practices.

5. Palliative Care Research :
Research in palliative care is essential to advancing the field. If you have an interest in research, you could move into research positions or take part in collaborative research projects.

6. Palliative Care Liaison Nurse :
The role of palliative care liaison nurse involves working with various medical teams to ensure seamless coordination of palliative care for hospitalised patients.

7. Palliative Care Social Worker :
If you have social work skills, you could consider specialising as a palliative care social worker, offering emotional and practical support to patients and their families.

8. Administration of Palliative Care Programmes :
Some nurses specialise in administering palliative care programmes, ensuring that patients receive the services and resources they need.

9. Continuing education :
Career development options also include pursuing your own continuing education by attending workshops, conferences and advanced training courses to keep abreast of the latest developments.

10. Leadership at Health Policy Level :
Some nurses are involved in advocacy and health policy initiatives to improve access to palliative care and influence political decisions.

Career development in palliative care offers a range of options to suit different aspirations and interests. By choosing the path you are passionate about, you can not only enrich your career, but also make a significant contribution to improving the quality of life of patients and their families at the end of life.

Chapter 11:
Future prospects Palliative Care

Foreseeable developments in palliative care

Integrating New Technologies into Palliative Care

The integration of new technologies into palliative care has the potential to transform the way healthcare professionals interact with patients, families and colleagues, while improving the quality of care provided. These technologies offer innovative solutions to the challenges of palliative care and enrich the experience of patients at the end of life. Here's how new technologies can be integrated into palliative care:

1. Telecare and teleconsultation :
Telecare and teleconsultations enable patients to receive palliative care remotely, reducing the need to travel and facilitating access to care, particularly for patients in an advanced stage of illness or those living in remote areas.

2. Virtual Communication Platforms :
Virtual communication platforms facilitate communication between patients, families and members of the medical team. This can include discussions about care plans, symptom management and psychological support.

3. Electronic Medical Records :
Electronic medical records centralise medical information and facilitate the coordination of care between the different members of the team. This ensures that all the necessary information is accessible in real time.

4. Symptom Management applications :
Mobile applications specific to palliative care allow patients to monitor and report their symptoms, enabling the medical team to provide a rapid and appropriate response.

5. Telemedicine for Pain Management :
Telemedicine can be used to adjust pain management protocols remotely, enabling healthcare professionals to monitor and personalise treatments in real time.

6. Virtual Paediatric Palliative Care :
New technologies can be used to provide virtual paediatric palliative care, offering ongoing support to children with serious illnesses and their families.

7. Virtual Reality for Pain Management :
Virtual reality can be used to distract patients from pain and discomfort, offering a non-pharmacological approach to pain management.

8. Online Education and Training :
Online education platforms give nurses access to training and resources to keep up to date with the latest advances and best practices.

9. Home monitoring devices :
Home monitoring devices enable patients' vital signs and symptoms to be tracked remotely, enabling rapid intervention if necessary.

10. Social Networks and Online Support Groups :
Social networks and online support groups provide a space for patients and families to share their experiences, find emotional support and connect with others going through similar situations.

The successful integration of new technologies into palliative care requires a considered and ethical approach. It is essential to ensure that patients and families feel comfortable with the use of these technologies and that their confidentiality and security are maintained. By harnessing the benefits of new technologies, healthcare professionals in palliative care can improve the quality of care while maintaining a valuable human link with patients and families at the end of life.

Evolution of Care Delivery Models
The rapid evolution of palliative care has led to a review of traditional models of care delivery to better meet the varied and complex needs of patients at the end of life and their families. Care delivery models are evolving to provide more personalised, patient-centred care tailored to different clinical situations. Here's how palliative care delivery models have evolved:

1. Palliative care at home :
The home palliative care delivery model emphasises patient comfort in familiar surroundings. Care teams travel to the

147

patient's home to provide medical, emotional and supportive care.

2. Hospital Palliative Care Units :
Hospital-based palliative care units provide a dedicated space for patients requiring advanced palliative care, where a multidisciplinary team can provide comprehensive care.

3. Paediatric palliative care :
Paediatric palliative care delivery models are tailored to the specific needs of children with serious illnesses, focusing on emotional support and family care.

4. Outpatient palliative care :
Ambulatory palliative care is designed for patients whose state of health allows them to live at home, but who require regular medical interventions, follow-up and treatment adjustments.

5. Consultative Palliative Care Teams :
Advisory palliative care teams work in collaboration with primary care teams to provide advice, recommendations and specialist support for the management of symptoms and complex issues.

6. Palliative care in long-term care establishments :
This model aims to provide palliative care to patients residing in long-term care facilities such as retirement homes, with an emphasis on comfort and quality of life.

7. Community Palliative Care :
Community palliative care involves working closely with healthcare professionals in the community to provide care for patients and families at the end of life.

8. Palliative Care Integrated into Curative Treatments :
In this model, palliative care is integrated from the very beginning of the diagnosis of the disease, in parallel with curative treatments, to ensure a balance between cure and comfort.

9. Value-based palliative care :
This model takes into account the patient's values and preferences to tailor care and treatment decisions to their personal goals.

10. Palliative Care in Home Health Care :
Palliative care can be integrated into home healthcare services, offering patients a combination of medical care and support in a familiar environment.

The evolution of palliative care delivery models reflects the diverse needs of patients and families at the end of life. By choosing the most appropriate model for each clinical situation and collaborating with patients, families and colleagues, nurses can ensure that each patient receives the highest quality care that respects their unique needs and preferences.

Adapting to Demographic and Social Change
Palliative care is facing complex challenges as a result of the demographic and social changes taking place worldwide. These changes include an ageing population, increasing cultural diversity and changes in patients' expectations at the end of life. To respond effectively to these challenges, palliative care healthcare professionals need to adapt their approaches and models of care delivery. Here's how adaptation to demographic and social change can be addressed in palliative care:

1. Population ageing :
As the population ages, the number of patients requiring palliative care is increasing. Palliative care healthcare professionals need to develop specific skills to manage the complex health problems associated with ageing, while taking into account the preferences and life goals of elderly patients.

2. Cultural diversity :
Palliative care must be adapted to the cultural values, beliefs and practices of patients and their families. Palliative care health professionals must be sensitive to cultural diversity and provide care that respects these differences.

3. Multidisciplinary and interprofessional approaches :
Demographic and social changes require a multidisciplinary and interprofessional approach to meet the complex needs of patients at the end of life. Palliative care teams need to work with a range of health professionals to provide holistic and comprehensive care.

4. Promoting patient self-determination :
With social changes, patient self-determination is increasingly valued. Palliative care professionals must encourage patients to take an active part in making decisions about their care and end of life.

5. Raising awareness of gender issues :
Gender sensitivity is essential in palliative care, as end-of-life experiences can vary according to gender. Healthcare professionals need to be aware of these differences and provide appropriate care.

6. Integration of Communication Technologies :
Social changes have led to an increasing use of communication technologies. Health professionals in palliative care need to

149

integrate these technologies to maintain communication with patients, families and colleagues.

7. Promotion of Continuing Education :

In the face of demographic and social change, palliative care healthcare professionals need to keep abreast of new trends, best practice and innovations in the field through continuing education.

8. Adaptation of training programmes :

Palliative care training programmes need to be adapted to include specific skills for dealing with the issues associated with demographic and social change.

By proactively adapting to demographic and social changes, palliative care healthcare professionals can ensure that patients and their families receive high-quality care that meets their unique needs, while reflecting society's emerging values and expectations.

Technological advances and current innovations

Using telemedicine for palliative care

The use of telemedicine in palliative care has emerged as an innovative response to overcoming geographical barriers, improving access to care and ensuring ongoing support for patients at the end of life and their families. Telemedicine, which encompasses remote consultations, home monitoring and virtual communication, offers new possibilities for providing quality care to patients who are unable to travel or who prefer to receive care in their home environment. Here's how telemedicine is being used in palliative care:

1. Remote consultations :

Remote consultations allow patients to discuss their symptoms, concerns and needs with healthcare professionals in real time, without having to physically travel to the clinic. This is particularly beneficial for patients who are too ill to travel.

2. Follow-up at home :

Telemedicine enables healthcare professionals to monitor patients' vital signs and symptoms at home. Connected medical devices can automatically transmit data to healthcare professionals, who can then intervene when necessary.

150

3. Symptom management :
Telemedicine allows patients to report their symptoms using mobile applications or dedicated online platforms. Health professionals can then adjust treatments on the basis of the information provided.

4. Virtual Psychological Support :
Telemedicine offers the possibility of providing virtual psychological support to patients and families, which can be particularly useful for managing anxiety, depression and other emotional problems at the end of life.

5. End of Life Discussions :
Telemedicine can facilitate discussions on end-of-life preferences and treatment decisions between patients, families and healthcare professionals, even if the parties are geographically distant.

6. Training and Education :
Telemedicine can be used to provide training and education sessions for patients and families on topics such as symptom management, palliative care at home and end-of-life care.

7. Interdisciplinary collaboration :
Telemedicine facilitates collaboration between the different members of the palliative care team, enabling an integrated and coherent approach to care.

8. Reducing geographical barriers :
Telemedicine enables patients living in remote or underserved areas to access high-quality palliative care without having to travel long distances.

However, it is important to note that telemedicine cannot completely replace face-to-face interaction and human presence. It must be used judiciously, taking into account patients' needs and preferences. Furthermore, data security and the confidentiality of medical information must be rigorously protected when using telemedicine. By judiciously integrating telemedicine into the provision of palliative care, healthcare professionals can improve access to care and offer ongoing support to patients at the end of life, wherever they may be.

Mobile Applications for Symptom Management
Mobile applications are playing an increasingly important role in the delivery of palliative care by providing patients and families with practical tools for managing symptoms, communicating with healthcare professionals and accessing useful information.

These applications are designed to improve the quality of life of patients at the end of life by enabling them to monitor their symptoms, receive personalised advice and be better prepared for the challenges they may face. Here's how mobile apps are being used for symptom management in palliative care:

1. Monitoring and follow-up of symptoms :
Mobile applications allow patients to track and monitor their symptoms on a daily basis, helping healthcare professionals to adjust treatments as the situation evolves.

2. Pain management :
Mobile applications can provide tools for monitoring and managing pain, such as pain rating scales, medication reminders and relaxation techniques.

3. Monitoring of side effects :
Patients can use apps to report the side effects of medicines and treatments, enabling healthcare professionals to take swift action.

4. Advice and recommendations :
Mobile apps often provide personalised advice for managing specific symptoms, which can help patients better understand their options and make informed decisions.

5. Virtual communication :
Some applications allow patients to communicate with healthcare professionals via secure messaging, making it easier to follow up regularly and deal with urgent matters.

6. Information on Palliative Care :
Mobile applications offer educational information on palliative care, treatment options, advance directives and other important topics.

7. Mood and well-being monitoring :
Apps can help patients monitor their mood and emotional well-being, enabling healthcare professionals to detect signs of depression or anxiety.

8. Personalised Care :
Mobile applications can tailor information and recommendations to individual patient needs and preferences.

9. Reminders and planning :
Mobile applications can help patients organise their medical appointments, medication and other aspects of their care plan.

10. Support for Relatives :
Some apps also offer resources and support for relatives of patients at the end of life, helping them to better understand palliative care and support the patient.

It is important to note that mobile applications for symptom management must be chosen carefully, ensuring their reliability, data security and user-friendliness. Healthcare professionals can play a role in educating patients on the appropriate use of these applications and in interpreting the data collected. The judicious use of mobile applications can improve patient autonomy and foster better communication between patients, their families and palliative care healthcare professionals.

Here are some examples of mobile applications designed to help with symptom management, particularly in the context of palliative care:

- **PalliApp:** This application offers a range of features for managing symptoms in palliative care. Patients can track their symptoms, record pain, fatigue, appetite and other factors. The app also allows users to take notes, record their care preferences and communicate with their care team.
- **MySymptoms:** Designed to track symptoms in a variety of medical contexts, this application allows palliative care patients to track and report their daily symptoms such as pain, nausea, fatigue, etc. The data recorded can be shared with healthcare professionals to help adjust treatment plans. Recorded data can be shared with healthcare professionals to help adjust treatment plans.
- **Calmerry:** This application focuses on emotional and psychological support. It offers online therapy sessions with mental health professionals, which can help palliative care patients manage stress, anxiety and difficult emotions.
- **Medisafe:** This app allows patients to track their medication and intake, which is particularly useful for those with complex medication regimes in palliative care. The app sends reminders to take medicines on time and offers functionality to share data with care providers.
- **Cancer.Net Mobile:** An application developed by the American Society of Clinical Oncology, it provides information on cancer, resources on palliative care and advice on managing the symptoms associated with cancer at the end of life.
- **CareZone:** This application helps patients to organise their lives by providing tools for tracking medication, scheduling medical appointments and recording

153

symptoms and side effects. It can also be used to share information with relatives and care providers.

- **GeriPal:** Although primarily aimed at healthcare professionals, this app provides information and resources on palliative and geriatric care, which can be useful for professionals and families involved in care.
- **PainScale:** This application is designed specifically to help patients monitor and manage their pain. It allows users to record their pain levels, track medication taken and obtain information on pain management.

It's important to note that the quality and effectiveness of apps can vary, so it's advisable to consult reviews, ratings and talk to healthcare professionals before choosing a specific app for symptom management in palliative care.

Integrating Artificial Intelligence into Palliative Care Practice
Artificial intelligence (AI) has made significant advances in many areas of medicine, including palliative care. Integrating AI into palliative care practice offers opportunities to improve clinical decision-making, symptom management, communication with patients and families, as well as optimising medical resources. Here's how AI is being used in palliative care practice:

1. Prediction of Patient Needs :
AI can analyse past and real-time medical data to predict a patient's future needs in terms of symptoms, treatments and care. This enables healthcare professionals to plan care proactively.

2. Symptom Management :
AI can help monitor the symptoms of patients at the end of their lives and offer recommendations for adjusting treatments based on the data collected.

3. Biomedical Data Analysis :
AI can rapidly analyse vast quantities of biomedical data to identify patterns and relevant information, helping healthcare professionals to make informed decisions.

4. Decision Support :
By analysing medical data and clinical evidence, AI can provide suggestions for appropriate treatments, helping healthcare professionals to make complex decisions.

5. Personalised Care :
AI can use personal data to tailor care plans to each patient's specific needs and preferences.

6. Communication assistance :
AI-powered chatbots can answer questions from patients and their families, providing basic information and directing some to healthcare professionals when more complex interactions are required.

7. Early detection of complications :
AI can identify early signs of complications or worsening of the disease, enabling faster, more targeted intervention.

8. Research Data Analysis :
AI can analyse medical research data to identify new treatment approaches or to inform evidence-based clinical practice.

9. Resource management :
AI can help optimise the use of medical resources by identifying staffing requirements, hospital bed availability and appointment schedules.

However, the integration of AI into palliative care raises ethical and practical considerations, particularly in terms of data protection and confidentiality. Furthermore, AI should not replace the human and empathetic relationship between patients and healthcare professionals. Instead, it should be used to complement and enhance existing palliative care. Healthcare professionals play a crucial role in supervising and interpreting the results produced by AI, taking into account the specific context and values of each patient.

Challenges and opportunities for future nurses

Meeting the growing needs of an ageing population
With increasing life expectancy and an ageing population, palliative care is playing an increasingly essential role in meeting the specific needs of older people at the end of life. The challenges associated with ageing, such as chronic illnesses, mobility problems and medical complications, require a holistic, patient-centred approach to ensure optimal quality of life right up to the end. Here's how palliative care meets the growing needs of an ageing population:

1. Chronic Disease Management :

Palliative care offers a comprehensive approach to managing the chronic illnesses associated with ageing, such as diabetes, heart disease and Alzheimer's disease. It aims to reduce symptoms, improve quality of life and maintain patient autonomy.

2. Pain and Fatigue Management :

Older people are more likely to experience pain and fatigue as a result of underlying health problems. Palliative care targets these symptoms to minimise their impact on quality of life.

3. Emotional Support :

Ageing can be accompanied by social isolation, loss and bereavement. Palliative care offers emotional support to elderly patients by addressing their psychological needs and helping to alleviate feelings of loneliness.

4. End-of-life planning :

Palliative care facilitates end-of-life planning by helping older people to make decisions about their wishes regarding treatment, care and advance directives.

5. Maintaining Dignity :

Palliative care recognises the importance of preserving the dignity of older people at the end of their lives, taking into account their values and personal preferences.

6. Support for Relatives :

Palliative care also supports the families and loved ones of elderly patients at the end of life, helping them to understand the specific needs of older people and providing resources to help them in their support role.

7. Access to Personalised Care :

Palliative care is designed to meet the unique needs of each elderly patient, taking into account their medical history, preferences and goals of care.

8. Open and Respectful Communication :

Palliative care encourages open and respectful communication with elderly patients, giving them the opportunity to express their concerns, wishes and worries.

9. Transition to Comfort Care :

Elderly people at the end of life sometimes have specific needs in terms of comfort care. Palliative care ensures that these needs are taken into account and adapted as the situation evolves.

Palliative care healthcare professionals play a crucial role in adapting care to the specific needs of older people at the end of life. By focusing on overall symptom management, emotional support and respect for life choices, palliative care helps to ensure that older people spend their final days in dignity and comfort.

Maintaining a Balance between Technology and Humanity

As technological advances transform the delivery of palliative care, it is essential to maintain a balance between the use of technology and the importance of the human aspect of this sensitive care. Integrating technology can improve efficiency, accuracy and access to care, but it is equally important to preserve the human aspects of the relationship between patients, families and healthcare professionals. Here's how to maintain that balance:

1. Technology as a Tool, Not a Replacement:

Technology should be seen as a tool to improve care, not as a substitute for human interaction. Healthcare professionals must remain emotionally engaged and empathetic, while using technology to support their decisions and actions.

2. Personalised Care :

Technology can help personalise care using medical data and patient preferences, but healthcare professionals must remain attentive to the unique aspects of each individual.

3. Sensitive communication :

While digital communication tools can be convenient, they should not replace face-to-face conversations where possible. Sensitive and emotional discussions are best conducted face-to-face to ensure patients and families feel supported and heard.

4. Emotional Support and Compassion :

Technology cannot reproduce human warmth, empathy and compassion. Healthcare professionals must maintain a physical and emotional presence to respond to the emotional needs of patients and families.

5. Respect for Cultural and Ethical Values :

Technology must be used with respect for the patient's cultural and ethical values. Healthcare professionals must take account of individual beliefs and ensure that technology does not conflict with these values.

6. Continuing education :

Healthcare professionals must be trained in the appropriate use of technology in palliative care, with an emphasis on ethics, confidentiality and respect for patients.

7. Regular assessment :
It is important to regularly evaluate the effectiveness of technology in the delivery of palliative care. Patients and families must be consulted to ensure that their emotional and physical needs are always taken into account.

8. Flexibility and adaptability :
Technology is evolving rapidly. Healthcare professionals must be ready to adapt to new technological solutions while maintaining a strong human commitment.

In summary, the use of technology in palliative care can offer many benefits, but it is imperative not to lose sight of the crucial human element of the care relationship. The balance between technology and humanity ensures that patients and families receive the attentive, empathetic and individualised care they need to face the end of life with dignity and comfort.

Plea for Better Recognition and Resources for Palliative Care

Palliative care plays a crucial role in providing quality end-of-life care, offering comfort, dignity and emotional support to patients and their families. However, despite its importance, palliative care is not always fully recognised or adequately supported in terms of financial and human resources. Effective advocacy is essential to improve the recognition of palliative care and ensure that the necessary resources are allocated to provide optimal care to those who need it. Here's how to advocate for better recognition and increased resources for palliative care:

1. Public awareness :
Advocacy starts with raising public awareness. It is important to share information about the benefits of palliative care, demystify misunderstandings and show how it improves quality of life at the end of life.

2. Education of healthcare professionals :
It is essential to educate healthcare professionals about the importance of palliative care and how to integrate these approaches into their practice. This helps to ensure that all patients receive appropriate palliative care when needed.

3. Policy development :
Advocacy can involve working with policy makers to develop health policies that support palliative care. This may include

guidelines on resource allocation and the integration of palliative care into health systems.

4. Data and evidence collection :
Gathering data and evidence on the effectiveness of palliative care is essential to demonstrate its positive impact on patients' quality of life and the reduction of long-term healthcare costs.

5. Working with Patient Groups and Families :
Working closely with patient groups, families and patient advocates can strengthen advocacy by giving a voice to those directly affected.

6. Media campaigns :
Targeted media campaigns can help raise awareness of the importance of palliative care and influence **public opinion and decision-makers.**

7. Collaboration with Health Organisations :
Working with health organisations, hospitals and medical institutions to promote the integration of palliative care into their practices can have a significant impact.

8. Participation in public debates :
Participating in debates and public discussions on end-of-life and healthcare helps to raise awareness of palliative care issues.

9. Advocacy for Financial Resources :
Advocacy should also include a request for an adequate allocation of financial resources for palliative care, including funding for staff, training and services.

By advocating greater recognition and resources for palliative care, we can help to improve the quality of life of patients at the end of life and ensure that everyone can live out their final days with dignity, comfort and respect for their personal values.

www.ingramcontent.com/pod-product-compliance
Lightning Source LLC
Chambersburg PA
CBHW072205290526
45794CB00004B/1664